Instructor's Manual to Accompany

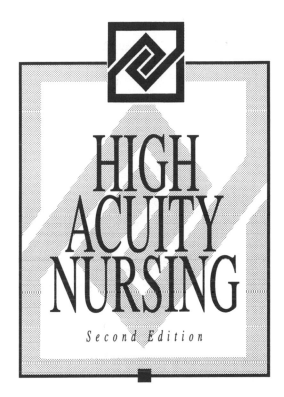

HIGH ACUITY NURSING

Second Edition

Pamela Stinson Kidd, RN, PhD, CEN, ARNP, FNP
Associate Professor
University of Kentucky College of Nursing
Lexington, Kentucky

Kathleen Dorman Wagner, RN, CS, MSN
Assistant Professor
University of Kentucky College of Nursing
Doctoral Student, College of Education
University of Kentucky
Lexington, Kentucky

APPLETON & LANGE
Stamford, CT

Copyright ©1997 by Appleton & Lange
A Simon & Schuster Company

97 98 99 00 01/ 10 9 8 7 6 5 4 3 2 1

Prentice Hall International (UK) Limited, London
Prentice Hall of Australia Pty. Limited, Sydney
Prentice Hall Canada, Inc., Toronto
Prentice Hall Hispanoamericana, S.A., Mexico
Prentice Hall of India Private Limited, New Delhi
Prentice Hall of Japan, Inc., Tokyo
Simon & Schuster Asia Pte. Ltd., Singapore
Editora Prentice Hall do Brasil Ltda., Rio de Janeiro
Prentice Hall, Upper Saddle River, New Jersey

ISBN 0-8385-3744-8

90000

9 780838 537442

ISBN 0-8385-3744-8

Acquisitions Editor: David P. Carroll

PRINTED IN THE UNITED STATES OF AMERICA

TABLE OF CONTENTS

PREFACE

PART I. PHYSIOLOGIC AND PSYCHOSOCIAL COMFORT

Take Home Cases (THC)
Acute Pain Management in the High Acuity Patient 3

Case Study
The Case of Mark Wade 11

PART II. RESPIRATION AND VENTILATION

Take Home Cases (THC)
Respiratory Process (Module 3) 21
Arterial Blood Gas Analysis (Module 4) 29
Mechanical Ventilation (Module 5) 39

Case Studies/Exercises
The Case of Pearl M 52
The Case of Thomas Bach 63
The Case of Raymond Sinclair 72
ABG Analysis Exercise 80

Problem Solving Exercise (PSE)
The Case of Marie M 82

Clinical Focus
Respiratory Process 92

PART III. CELLULAR OXYGENATION

Take Home Cases (THC)
Cellular Oxygenation (Module 7) 99
Shock States (Module 8) 101

Case Studies/Exercises
The Case of Mr. Jones *post·op* 103
The Case of Nancy T. 107

Clinical Focus
Cellular Oxygenation 110

PART IV. PERFUSION

Take Home Cases (THC)
Perfusion (Module 11) 115
Hemodynamic Monitoring (Module 12) 120
Electrocardiographic Monitoring and Related Cardiac Medications (Module 13) 123

Case Studies/Exercises
    The Case of Hugh Neff 124
    The Case of Mike Brown 130
    Hemodynamic Parameter Practice Sheet 133

Clinical Focus: Perfusion 135

PART V. NEUROLOGIC

Take Home Cases (THC)
    Responsiveness (Module 15) 141

Case Studies/Exercises
    The Case of Billy Bob 144
    The Case of Susan 149

Problem Solving Exercise (PSE)
    The Case of Mary Burns 153

PART VI. METABOLISM

Take Home Cases (THC)
    Metabolic Responses (Module 20) 165
    Altered Immune Function (Module 21) 176
    Acute Hepatic Dysfunction (Module 23) 187
    Altered Glucose Metabolism (Module 24) 195
    Acute Renal Dysfunction (Module 26) 205

Case Studies/Exercises
    Diabetic Crises Cases 213
    Immunocompetence Cases 225
    The Case of Joan T. 237
    The Case of C.R. Cramer (see also PSE version) 242
    The Case of Bob White 252

Problem Solving Exercise (PSE)
    The Case of C.R. Cramer (see also Case Study version) 260

Clinical Foci
    Endocrine Problems *do for clinical* 265
    Acute GI Problems *" " " pancreatitis / cirrhosis* 268

PART VII. INJURY

Take Home Cases (THC)
    Complex Wound Management (Module 28) 273
    Acute Burn Injury (Module 29) 275

Case Studies/Exercises
    The Case of Mary Mole *post-op / diabetes / wound* 278
    The Case of Bobby W. 282

Problem Solving Exercise (PSE)
    The Case of Mike Brady 293

Clinical Focus
    Injury   299

PART VIII. LIFE SPAN: SPECIAL NEEDS

Take Home Cases (THC)
    The Acutely Ill Pediatric Patient (Module 32)   303
    The Acutely Ill Obstetric Patient (Module 33)   306
    The Acutely Ill Elderly Patient (Module 34)   309

Case Studies/Exercises
    The Case of Mary Case   311
    The Case of Baby TJ   318
    The Case of Amanda   325

OVERHEAD TRANSPARENCY MASTERS   327

Instructor Manual for High Acuity Nursing

The purpose of this manual is to facilitate application of **High Acuity Nursing** in the classroom. The book's self study format decreases the need to spend valuable class time focusing on review of previously learned concepts. The modules encourage the student, rather than the instructor, to synthesize. Instructor time can be used to implement case studies, problem based learning exercises, and reality based scenarios that require the student to apply this synthesis in a variety of patient care situations.

We use **High Acuity Nursing** as the required text in our Senior Adult II nursing course. The classroom portion of this course consists of two components:
1. pre-class preparation - self study modules
2. classroom activities - Concept clarification, nursing management and application and analysis of case studies

In addition, we have developed a variety of clinical foci that help reinforce some of the classroom material.

Pre-class Preparation - Self Study Modules

Self directed study focuses on adult learning principles, placing the responsibility on the learner for mastery of content. Every seminar focuses learning by presenting a single concept. It is a course expectation that students will read (or at least scan) the appropriate module/s prior to class. Module material is not necessarily covered in class. This allows redirecting of educational energies and resources towards application of module principles and problem solving exercises using the nursing process.

Take Home Cases (THCs) have been developed for many of the modules. Our students have indicated that THCs assist them in focusing on critical module information during reading. One useful strategy is to have students turn in the THC at the beginning of class (they are not accepted after class). Each THC is graded, either for content, or based on whether it was turned in. Our THCs are all weighted the same (either 5 or 10 points works well). We have a bulletin board on which we stick the case "key" after class so that students can look at (or copy) the answer. If faculty has the time to actually grade content, they can be very enlightening as to what each student actually comprehends. They can also be provided to students to use as enrichment.

Classroom Activities

Concept Clarification, Nursing Management, and Application

We suggest that class time be structured yet interactive. Difficult module concepts may be focused on and nursing management discussed as delineated. The emphasis is placed on nursing assessment and interventions, major nursing diagnoses related to the topic, major diagnostic testing appropriate to the concept, and evaluation of patient outcomes.

Class - Application and Analysis of Case Studies

Ideally, the majority of each class session is used for reality based case analysis and problem solving exercises. In this manual are multiple exercises provided for most major parts of the book. Additional learning tools are provided such as ABG and hemodynamic trend analysis worksheets. Time will probably not allow you to implement each of the cases provided. We encourage you to try them. We have found that they sharpen students' critical thinking skills. Work may be performed individually or in small groups. We have used them in groups as large as sixty and as small as three. Ideally, small group learning should consist of groups of ten or less. The learning exercises require use of nursing inference and critical thinking skills. Case studies and exercises have taken many hours to develop. If you decide to use them, the authors ask that you include the provided author & text identification.

As an instructor, it is suggested that you read each module to help you in deciding which case studies and exercises to select or modify. You will find that many of the case studies and problem solving exercises are appropriate to enrich classroom teaching in more than one module. This is because the majority of the cases have been developed from real case scenarios where multisystem dysfunction is the mainstream.

Examples include: The Case of C.R. Cramer, which focuses on nutrition and immunocompetence; The Case of Mary Burns addresses brain attack (CVA) and nutrition; and The Case of Bobby W. relates to acute burn injury, immunocompetence, and nutrition.

Class Content Support Activities: Clinical Foci

Over the years, we have developed clinical foci for many of the topics of the text. These activities focus primarily on clinical assessment of the patient with a particular problem. They also contain nursing process activities for the student to complete based on the newly collected database. We have found that during clinicals, students do well to complete the clinical assessments. We either have students complete the remainder of the focus on their own and turn the completed form in to the instructor, or we use the nursing process portion of the Clinical Focus as the topic for our post-conference discussion.

Thank you for supporting our book!

Pamela Kidd

Kathleen Wagner

PART I

PHYSIOLOGIC AND PSYCHOSOCIAL COMFORT

Part I.   Table of Contents

PART I. PHYSIOLOGIC AND PSYCHOSOCIAL COMFORT

Take Home Case (THC)

Acute Pain Management in the High Acuity Patient (Module 2)   3

Case Study

The Case of Mark Wade   11

TAKE HOME CASE
Module 2: Acute Pain Management in the High Acuity Patient

DIRECTIONS

In narrative form, complete the following questions or statements based on the Module reading assignment. To better comprehend this material, it is best to answer the items in your own words rather than copying answers from the text. By doing so, you can evaluate what you actually understand.

READING ASSIGNMENT: *High Acuity Nursing, 2nd ed.* -- Module 2: Acute Pain Management in the High Acuity Patient
****

SITUATION: Andrea P. a 43 year old woman, fell asleep while driving home from her night shift job. Her car drove off of the road and hit a tree at a speed of about 45 miles per hour. Andrea sustained multiple injuries including: a head injury, a liver laceration, and multiple bone fractures. She has been in the trauma intensive care unit for four days.

SECTION ONE: PHYSIOLOGY – A REVIEW

Andrea indicates that she is experiencing pain.

1. What is the difference between somatic and visceral pain?

2. Which type(s) of pain is Andrea most likely experiencing?

3. Pain receptors are one type of _____ receptor. Pain receptors are also called _____. The function of pain receptors is_____.

4. "A" type pain fibers differ from C fibers in what ways?

5. Andrea's body is releasing certain chemical mediators that influence pain. What effect do enkephalins and endorphins have on Andrea's pain?

SECTION TWO: THE MULTIFACETED NATURE OF PAIN

6. How does the focus differ between the definitions of pain as stated by McCaffery and AHCPR?

7. Which type(s) of acute pain is Andrea most likely experiencing? Why?

⑨ According to the Loeser and Cousins model of pain, the nurse can only objectively measure which facet?

10. To activate the pain response, noxious stimuli must exist in sufficient quantities to:

Andrea is experiencing severe pain. Could she be suffering, as well?

⑪ How does suffering differ from pain? Can we measure suffering?

⑫ What is the difference between pain expressing and pain controlling behaviors? (Include examples of both)

SECTION THREE: ACUTE PAIN IN THE HIGH ACUITY PATIENT

Andrea is currently on bed rest. She has a pin below her left knee which is attached to traction. She has an abdominal incision resulting from an exploratory laparotomy and splenectomy. She has an endotracheal tube in place, a small bore feeding tube in her left nostril and a Salem sump tube in her right nostril. She is requiring endotracheal suctioning every one to two hours. She is in a trauma ICU and is attached to a cardiac monitor and mechanical ventilator. She has a central intravenous line in her right subclavian vein and a left radial arterial line.

⑬ Based on what you know about Andrea, list her potential sources of pain:

14. Briefly explain in what way pain is affected by stress:

SECTION FOUR: PAIN ASSESSMENT

You are about to assess Andrea for pain.

⑮ Since Andrea cannot verbally tell you about her pain, how will you perform a pain assessment?

16. When would the nurse consider using a multidimensional scale?

17. If Andrea is unable to assist with any type of self-assessment, what strategies can the nurse use to assess for the presence of pain? Can the nurse write down a pain intensity level based on nursing observations?

SECTION FIVE: MANAGEMENT OF ACUTE PAIN

18. Describe the purpose of the WHO Analgesic Ladder:

19. The nurse has been working throughout the shift trying to control Andrea's pain but has been unable to do so. She has been receiving analgesic therapy for the mild pain without sufficient relief. Explain the appropriate response to this situation according to the WHO Analgesic Ladder:

20. After major surgery, AHCPR recommends use of the _____ route to administer analgesics. Briefly explain why:

21. What are the advantages of patient controlled analgesia (PCA)?

22. List the three AHCPR guidelines for use of nonpharmacologic interventions that best apply to high acuity patients:

SECTION SIX: ISSUES IN INADEQUATE TREATMENT OF ACUTE PAIN

23. Assuming Andrea requires opioid therapy for an extended period of time, she will definitely develop some degree of which of the following opioid related problems: tolerance, physical dependence, psychologic dependence (addiction), or opioid pseudoaddiction?

24. Explain the meaning of "opiophobia":

25. One of your co-workers confides in you that she is afraid to administer any more opioid to Andrea because of potential respiratory depression. What can you tell her that may lessen her concern?

26. Briefly explain the preventive approach to pain management:

27. If the titration approach to pain management is used, the goal of therapy is

28. List the factors the clinician needs to consider when using the titration approach:

    1.

    2.

    3.

    4.

SECTION SEVEN: PAIN MANAGEMENT IN SPECIFIC PATIENT POPULATIONS

29. If Andrea were elderly, the nurse would need to take the effects of aging into consideration when managing her acute pain. List at least 3 effects of aging relevant to drug therapy:

30. What are the implications of concurrent organ dysfunction (liver and/or kidney) on pain management?

Case Study
The Case of Mark Wade

You are the nurse assigned to Mark Wade, 69 years old, a transfer patient who was flown to your facility for admission into the coronary care unit. You have just been informed that Mr. Wade has arrived and is placed in his bed.

Recent History

Approximately six weeks ago, Mr. Wade developed anorexia, increased dyspepsia with fullness and increased gas. The symptoms did not increase with eating but caused him to eat less. Three to four days ago, he developed increased shortness of breath with paroxysmal nocturnal dyspnea (PND) and increased peripheral edema. At this time, his wife took him to the local hospital's emergency department (ED). X-ray showed effusion, vascular congestion, and cardiomegaly. His EKG showed signs of an old diaphragmatic infarction with marked lateral wall S-T abnormalities. Mr. Wade complained that he had been steadily losing weight but that the "swelling" was hiding this loss. He indicated that according to his scales, he had gained six pounds overnight without eating much salt. Because of his signs and symptoms, he was admitted to the ICU. This morning his urine output dropped, his blood pressure increased, and his arterial blood gases worsened. At that time he was air lifted to your facility.

Past History

Mr. Wade is a retired miner. He developed arteriosclerotic heart disease with angina five years ago. He required a triple coronary bypass graft a year later. Last year he sustained a myocardial infarction and has had unstable angina since that time. Mr. Wade has a long history of pneumoconiosis (Black Lung Disease) and diabetes mellitus. He has been on the following medications at home: Glyburide, Nitro patch, Digoxin, Lasix, Slow-K, Apresoline, and Verapamil. He has no known allergies.

The Initial Appraisal

Upon walking into his room for the first time you quickly note the following:

General appearance: Mr. Wade is an elderly caucasian male. He is bald. His face is pale but pink and diaphoretic. He coughs frequently with frothy sputum. He is wearing glasses. He is connected to the cardiac monitor which shows a sinus rhythm with occasional premature ventricular contractions. His pulse is 96 and his oxygen saturation is 90%.

Signs of distress: You note that Mr. Wade's breathing is labored. His respirations are loud and moist. He is confused and lethargic but moves all extremities appropriately upon command and stimulation.

Other: Mr. Wade has an IV of 5% Dextrose and 0.45 Normal Saline infusing through a peripheral line in his left hand.

Systemic Bedside Assessment

Head and Neck
Mr. Wade is oriented to person and place only. His Glasgow Coma Scale score is 14. He is moderately hard of hearing. His neck veins are distended with the HOB at 45 degrees.

Chest
Pulmonary status: Bilateral rhonchi and crackles (rales) are heard throughout his lung fields.
Cardiac status: S_1 and S_2 are auscultated with a loud S_4. ECG pattern shows sinus tachycardia with occasional PVC.

Abdomen

Bowel sounds are hypoactive. He complains of tenderness in the right upper quadrant. His abdomen is distended and tight in the lower quadrants which prove to be tympanic on percussion.

Pelvis

A urinary catheter is in place, draining a small amount of dark yellow urine. After checking the nurses notes from the referring facility, you note that his output has been 80cc in six hours. He has no bladder distention.

Extremities:

+1 peripheral pulses are assessed. His capillary refill is less than three seconds. Nail beds are pale-pink. Moderate (3+) pitting edema is noted in all extremities. His skin is warm, clammy, and taut.

Posterior:

Sacral edema is present. No signs of skin breakdown are noted. Several reddened areas are noted over the mid-back. Posterior lung field auscultation is performed and rales and rhonchi are noted throughout the posterior fields, louder than the anterior assessment.

Vital Signs:

Currently: BP = 140/88; P = 96, regular; R = 28/minute, labored; T = 98.8
His ranges over the past 48 hours:
BP = $\underline{160 - 120}$, P = 90 - 120/minute, R = 20 - 30/minute, T = 97.0 - 99.4
     92 - 88

Psychosocial Assessment:

Mr. Wade was the "breadwinner" of the family until his MI last year. Prior to that time he had been able to control his angina with nitroglycerin sufficiently to keep him in the workforce. Mrs. Wade worked as a mail carrier but had to quit two months ago to care for Mr. Wade when his condition made him housebound.

Mrs. Wade indicates that the family is a very close unit and has stayed together very well throughout Mr. Wade's illness. She also states that they have very strong religious beliefs and that this factor has been helpful. When asked of specific concerns about Mr. Wade's admission she states that she does not believe that her husband will live to return home. Her two daughters live a short distance from Mr. and Mrs. Wade, and approximately 100 miles from the facility.

Mr. Wade receives a variety of income from the following sources: 1) Social Security; 2) Black Lung Benefits; and 3) United Mine Worker Pension Fund.

Six Hours Post Coronary Care Unit Admission:

Mr. Wade's condition continues to deteriorate. He is more lethargic and only responds to painful stimuli. He has had the following ECG changes: S-T elevation with an increasing amount of unifocal PVCs. He is made NPO. His diagnostic data is as follows:

Significant Labs and other tests:

SERUM:

WBC with diff.: WBC = 14.2, Segs = 9500, Bands = 3100, Lymphs = 1000.
RBC: 4.14
Glucose = 285
BUN = 75, Creatinine = 2.2,   Uric acid = 8.9
Electrolytes: Within normal ranges except for: Potassium = 2.9; Sodium = 123; Chloride = 76
Digoxin Level = 2.2

SPUTUM:
  Hemophilus.
PORTABLE CHEST X-RAY:
  Bilateral pleural effusions noted with cardiomegaly.

INTAKE AND OUTPUT:
  Last 24 hours: I = 2150 mL and O = 955 mL
WEIGHT:
  Admission = 196 pounds. Last week = 180 pounds.   Most Current = 166 pounds
ARTERIAL BLOOD GASES:
  On 2 liters of oxygen nasal cannula: pH = 7.48, $PaCO_2$ = 30, PaO_2 = 50, HCO_3 = 30, SpO_2 = 80%.

You and the physician approach the family to tell them that Mr. Wade will require intubation and mechanical ventilation as well as dialysis. Mrs. Wade asks, "Is he ever going home?". One of Mrs. Wade's daughters, who has since arrived states, "Oh Momma, you can't let daddy go yet".

The Respiratory Therapist pulls you aside and tells you that all of the ventilators in house are in use. He has called his supervisor to arrange to get additional back up units. If Mr. Wade is intubated, one of two options are available. Someone else could be weaned early or Mr. Wade can be "bagged" until the additional unit arrives. Both the respiratory therapy department and the coronary care unit are short staffed on this shift.

The Case of Mark Wade: Study Guide

Admitting Nursing Diagnoses:_____

Age:_____

Note: The Case of Mark Wade is a reality based case presentation. The data available may show evidence of multiple problem areas. The focus of today's case study, however, is the psychosocial issues surrounding his care. Thus, most of the questions in this exercise will center around consideration of these issues.

1.   **Past Medical and Social History:**

2.   **Events leading to admission:**

3.   **Initial Appraisal**
        What abnormal data did you collect from your initial appraisal of Mark?
        What is the significance of this data?

4.   **Based on your initial appraisal, what priority assessments will you immediately focus on?**
        1st priority?

        2nd priority?

5.   **Psychosocial Assessment**
        a.   Although typically applied to patients, family members also proceed through the stages of the patient's illness. What stage of illness does Mrs. Wade appear to be going through based on her response to the physician's clinical update?

        b.   What strategies can the nurse use to assist with family coping?

        c.   What environmental stressors is Mr. Wade exposed to because of his critical status and the hospital environment?

        d.   What actions can the nurse take to decrease environmental stressors?

6.   **Cluster the data to reflect three psychosocial considerations in Mr. Wade's case.**

        CLUSTER #1: Family Grieving

CLUSTER #2: Need for Family Coping

CLUSTER #3: Need for Spiritual Resources

CLUSTER #4: Difficulty Making Treatment Decisions

7. **Based on your data clusters/problems, what do you see as your priority nursing diagnoses?**
    Focus on his respiratory status.

8. **List appropriate <u>independent</u> nursing interventions that address the nursing diagnoses you have chosen.**

    1.

    2.

    3.

    4.

    5.

    6.

    7.

If time allows, consider the following group activity:

9. Analyze the dilemma of putting Mr. Wade on the ventilator and initiating dialysis. Don't expect to agree on all of the points of the analysis. You need to listen, recognize, and tolerate the differences of opinion that are a natural occurrence when a true dilemma exists.

    A. Identify the facts present and missing.
    B. Identify facts easily obtained.
    C. Identify facts difficult to obtain.
    D. Identify why the situation involves an ethical conflict.
    E. Identify solutions to the conflict.
    F. Identify the values promoted or sacrificed by each of the identified options.
    G. Relate your personal value system (as delineated in the value clarification exercise) to the solution/s.
    H. Explain why some values are best sacrificed or promoted in the situation. (justify the group's value judgment).

The Case of Mark Wade Study Guide
Instructor Guide

Admitting Nursing Diagnoses:_____

Age:_____

Note: The Case of Mark Wade is a reality based case presentation. The data available may show evidence of multiple problem areas. The focus of today's case study, however, is the psychosocial issues surrounding his care. Thus, most of the questions in this exercise will center around consideration of these issues.

_____

1.   **Past Medical and Social History:**
        Black Lung Disease
        Diabetes
        MI, post triple coronary bypass, previous breadwinner quit work because of health

2.   **Events leading to admission:**
        increasing dyspnea
        increasing weight gain

3.   **Initial Appraisal**
        What abnormal data did you collect from your initial appraisal of Mark?
        dyspnea, frothy sputum, PVCs, wet respirations,
        What is the significance of this data?
        Indicates left heart failure

4.   **Based on your initial appraisal, what priority assessments will you immediately focus in on?**
        1st priority?
        Ventilation/Respiratory
        2nd priority?
        Perfusion/Cardiac

5.   **Psychosocial Assessment**
        a.   Although typically applied to patients, family members also proceed through the stages of the patient's illness. What stage of illness does Mrs. Wade appear to be going through based on her response to the physician's clinical update? *(restitution)*

        b.   What strategies can the nurse use to assist with family coping? *(build communication, assist with problem solving, offer hospital resources, connect with community resources)*

        c.   What environmental stressors is Mr. Wade exposed to because of his critical status and the hospital environment? *(restricted movement, cardiac monitor noise, increased lighting, decreased privacy, decreased rest periods, lack of olfactory and gustatory stimulation due to his NPO status)*

        d.   What actions can the nurse take to decrease environmental stressors? *(dim lights, ROM, cluster interventions to allow uninterrupted rest, mouth care)*

6.   **Cluster the data to reflect three psychosocial considerations in Mr. Wade's case.**

        CLUSTER #1: Family Grieving
        Wife does not believe husband will live to go home from the hospital
        Patient responds only to painful stimuli

        CLUSTER #2: Need for Family Coping
        Wife quit work 2 months ago to care for husband
        Patient's prognosis is poor

CLUSTER #3: Need for Spiritual Resources
Family has to make a decision regarding degree of life support to initiate
Strong religious beliefs that have facilitated coping in the past

CLUSTER #4: Difficulty Making Treatment Decisions
Daughter ambivalent about her father's treatment. Wants to save daddy and place him on ventilator.
Mother/wife wants to know husband's prognosis before making decision. May produce family conflict.

7. **Based on your data clusters/problems, what do you see as your priority nursing diagnoses?**
Focus on his respiratory status.

1. _____**Family Coping: Potential for Growth R/T** *patient's deterioration.* _____.
   The family will effectively cope with Mr. Wade's physical status, as evidenced by:
   a) *family making collaborative decision*
   b) *discusses plans for life after patient's death*
   c) *family is able to communicate effectively with one another and with staff*

2. _____**Decisional Conflict R/T** *intubation decision* _____.
   The family will demonstrate effective decision making, as evidenced by:
   a) *collecting data and facts about patient's condition*
   b) *asking for assistance as needed in processing information*
   c) *making a decision and not changing the decision*
   d) *not regretting choice made*

3. _____**Anticipatory Grieving R/T** *patient's prognosis* _____.
   The family will effectively grieve, as evidenced by:
   a) *showing emotions*
   b) *verbally expressing goodbyes*
   c) *speaking of things they will miss about patient*

4. _____**Spiritual Distress R/T** *religious beliefs regarding death* _____.
   The patient and family will support their belief system, as evidenced by:
   a) *prayer*
   b) *using symbols of their religion as appropriate*
   c) *incorporating their religion in planning for patient's funeral*

8. **List appropriate _independent_ nursing interventions that address the nursing diagnoses you have chosen.**

   1. Refer to chaplain/religious resource person
   2. Assist family to discuss choices by providing information and setting for discussion
   3. Treat patient with dignity and maintain comfort care
   4. Include family and religious customs in caregiving
   5. Encourage family to talk with patient, keep family at bedside
   6. Encourage family to share memories of patient

   If time allows, consider the following group activity:

9. Analyze the dilemma of putting Mr. Wade on the ventilator and initiating dialysis. Don't expect to agree on all of the points of the analysis. You need to listen, recognize, and tolerate the differences of opinion that are a natural occurrence when a true dilemma exists.

   A. Identify the facts present and missing.
   B. Identify facts easily obtained.
   C. Identify facts difficult to obtain.

D. Identify why the situation involves an ethical conflict.

E. Identify solutions to the conflict.

F. Identify the values promoted or sacrificed by each of the identified options.

G. Relate your personal value system (as delineated in the value clarification exercise) to the solution/s.

H. Explain why some values are best sacrificed or promoted in the situation. (justify the group's value judgment).

PART II

RESPIRATION AND VENTILATION

Part II. Table of Contents

PART II: RESPIRATION AND VENTILATION

Take Home Cases (THC)
  Respiratory Process (Module 3)   21
  Arterial Blood Gas Analysis (Module 4)   29
  Mechanical Ventilation (Module 5)   39

Case Studies / Exercises
  The Case of Pearl M.   52
  The Case of Thomas Bach   63
  The Case of Raymond Sinclair   72
  ABG Analysis Exercise   79

Problem Solving Exercise (PSE): The Case of Marie M.   82

Clinical Focus: Respiratory Process   92

Take Home Case
Module 3: Respiratory Process

DIRECTIONS

Complete the following questions or statements based on the Module reading assignment. To better comprehend this material, it is best to answer the items in your own words rather than copying answers from the text. By doing so, you can evaluate what you actually understand.

READING ASSIGNMENT: *High Acuity Nursing, 2nd ed.* -- Module 3: Respiratory Process
****

SITUATION: Thomas E. is a 16 year old high school student who has been admitted to the hospital in acute respiratory distress. He is diagnosed as having acute bacterial pneumonia in his right lower lobe.

SECTION ONE: VENTILATION

1. Tom's lung compliance has decreased. Briefly explain how reduced compliance will effect his ventilatory status.

SECTION TWO: DIFFUSION

2. Briefly explain how a condition such as bacterial pneumonia can interfere with two factors associated with diffusion, surface area and thickness.

    Surface Area:

    Thickness:

SECTION THREE: VENTILATION - PERFUSION RELATIONSHIP

3. Explain in what way and why turning Tom to his affected (right) side could affect his oxygenation status based on the ventilation-perfusion relationship.

SECTION FOUR: RIGHT - TO - LEFT SHUNT

4. Tom develops hypoxemia that responds well to supplemental oxygen. Based on the concept of right-to-left shunt, state the type of shunt Tom is experiencing and briefly explain in what way this type of shunt is different from the other forms of shunt.

SECTION FIVE: PULMONARY FUNCTION EVALUATION

5. Tom weighs 56.8 kg. His normal tidal volume should range from _____ to _____ mL.

    The nurse would become concerned if his tidal volume dropped to below _____ mL which would reflect development of hypoventilation.

6. Tom's tidal volume is currently 400 mL and his respiratory rate is 40 breaths per minute. Based on the above data, his minute ventilation would be _____ L/minute. Briefly explain the significance of his current minute ventilation:

SECTION SIX: RESTRICTIVE VS OBSTRUCTIVE PULMONARY DISORDERS

7. Briefly explain how Tom's pneumonia meets the criteria for a restrictive pulmonary disease.

8. Tom has a long history of asthma. Asthma is a(n) restrictive / obstructive (circle one) disease process?

9. If Tom has an acute asthmatic episode, explain how his pulmonary tree would be affected.

10. Tom has an uncle, whose name is Henry. Henry was diagnosed with chronic bronchitis and emphysema ten years ago. On Henry's latest chest x-ray, it was noted that he had evidence of *cor pulmonale*.

    Briefly explain what cor pulmonale is.

    Describe the significance of this pulmonary complication to Uncle Henry's long term health outcomes.

SECTION SEVEN: ACUTE RESPIRATORY FAILURE

11. During his hospital stay, Tom develops acute respiratory failure. Briefly differentiate respiratory failure from respiratory insufficiency.

12. In your own words, define acute (adult) respiratory distress syndrome (ARDS).

13. Tom has been developing increasing symptoms of hypoxemia throughout the day. The physician orders oxygen therapy. If Tom has developed ARDS, the nurse would anticipate that his oxygen therapy would have what effect on his oxygenation status?

14. Tom's latest PaO_2 on 100 % oxygen therapy is 58 mm Hg. According to Table 3-8, what can be said about his PaO_2?

SECTION EIGHT: RESPIRATORY ASSESSMENT

15. Briefly explain why the nurse should obtain a nutritional history from Tom.

16. The nurse should assess Tom for the three most common complaints associated with pulmonary disorders. These include:

    1.

    2.

    3.

17. Tom is complaining of shortness of breath. The nurse charts that he is dyspneic. Dyspnea is a(n) subjective / objective (circle one) term. It is associated with increased _____.

18. Tom is complaining of chest pain. If his description of the pain he is experiencing is typical of pleuritic pain, you would expect to describe in as

19. Tom is coughing up secretions. In the absence of infection, Tom's secretions should have what appearance?

20. You are auscultating Tom's chest. When you place your stethoscope over the area of his pneumonia, you would probably hear what types of adventitious breath sounds?

SECTION NINE: RESPIRATORY CALCULATIONS

21. The Ideal Alveolar Gas Equation is a method of measuring what respiratory related gas factor?

22. Which of the respiratory calculations helps to estimate shunt? Which is considered least accurate?

SECTION TEN: DEVELOPING A PULMONARY PLAN OF CARE

23. Assuming that the nurse needs to configure a plan of care using nursing diagnoses, which respiratory related nursing diagnosis focuses on the rate, rhythm and depth of breathing?

24. You have just written the nursing diagnosis, *Impaired gas exchange*. What would be the most appropriate expected patient outcomes to measure this diagnosis?

25. After assessing Tom's respiratory status, you write the nursing diagnosis: *Ineffective airway clearance*. List at least 5 nursing interventions that would be appropriate to include on the plan of care:

    1.

    2.

    3.

    4.

Take Home Case
Respiratory Process
Instructor Guide

DIRECTIONS

In narrative form, complete the following questions or statements based on the Module reading assignment.

READING ASSIGNMENT: *High Acuity Nursing, 2ⁿᵈ ed.* -- Module 3: Respiratory Process
****

SITUATION: Thomas E. is a 16 year old high school student who has been admitted to the hospital in acute respiratory distress. He is diagnosed as having acute bacterial pneumonia in his right lower lobe.

SECTION ONE: VENTILATION

1.	Tom's lung compliance has decreased. Briefly explain how reduced compliance will effect his ventilatory status.
	ANSWER: As the lungs become more still due to decreasing compliance, Tom will experience an increase in work of breathing and decreased tidal volumes which places him at risk for problems associated with hypoventilation.

SECTION TWO: DIFFUSION

2.	Briefly explain how a condition such as bacterial pneumonia can interfere with two factors associated with diffusion, surface area and thickness.

	Surface Area: *Conditions such as pneumonia can decrease surface area by partially or completely obstructing alveoli with exudate from the infective process. In addition, if he is experiencing pleuritic pain, he may develop atelectasis due to hypoventilation. Atelectasis also decreases surface area.*

	Thickness: *Pneumonia is associated with an inflammatory response which causes edema, thereby thickening the alveolar-capillary membrane.*

SECTION THREE: VENTILATION - PERFUSION RELATIONSHIP

3.	Explain in what way and why turning Tom to his affected (right) side could affect his oxygenation status based on the ventilation-perfusion relationship.
	ANSWER: Turning Tom to his affected side could cause hypoxemia. Since gas flows through the path of least resistance and is not gravity dependent, more air will move into his left lung, which is not infected and is positioned higher than the right lung -- this leads to reduced ventilation to the affected lung. Since blood is gravity dependent, it will have a natural tendency to increase flow to the dependent lung, which, since Tom is laying on his right side, will be the right lung. This will cause more blood to be in the right lung than in the left. The end result is a mismatching of ventilation and perfusion. Right lung now has low ventilation in relation to perfusion.

SECTION FOUR: RIGHT - TO - LEFT SHUNT

4.	om develops hypoxemia that responds well to supplemental oxygen. Based on the concept of right-to-left shunt, state the type of shunt Tom is experiencing and briefly explain in what way this type of shunt is different from the other forms of shunt.
	ANSWER: Tom is experiencing shunt like effect. This problem differs from the other forms of shunt in that with shunt like effect, the alveoli are not completely bypassed during gas exchange; whereas, with anatomic shunt and capillary shunt, involved alveoli do not take part in gas exchange at all. With shunt like effect, perfusion is in excess of ventilation due to decreased ventilation or a diffusion defect

SECTION FIVE: PULMONARY FUNCTION EVALUATION

5. Tom weighs 56.8 kg. His normal tidal volume should range from _____ to _____ mL.

    The nurse would become concerned if his tidal volume dropped to below _____ mL which would reflect development of hypoventilation.

    ANSWERS: 398 mL to 511 mL; 227 mL.

6. Tom's tidal volume is currently 400 and his respiratory rate is 40 breaths per minute. Based on the above data, his minute ventilation would be _____ L/minute. Briefly explain the significance of his current minute ventilation.

    ANSWER: 16 L/minute. A sustained minute ventilation over 10 l/minute reflects a significantly increased work of breathing. As Tom become exhausted, he is at high risk for development of ventilatory insufficiency or failure (hypoventilation).

SECTION SIX: RESTRICTIVE VS OBSTRUCTIVE PULMONARY DISORDERS

7. Briefly explain how Tom's pneumonia meets the criteria for a restrictive pulmonary disease.
    ANSWER: Tom's pneumonia has decreased the number of functioning alveoli. His lungs are less compliant, thus he cannot get volume into his lung which will decrease his TLC (total lung capacity) but he can move air out of his lungs. His problems with hypoxemia are also typical of severe restrictive pulmonary problems.

8. Tom has a long history of asthma. Asthma is a(n) restrictive / ***obstructive*** (circle one) disease process.

9. If Tom has an acute asthmatic episode, explain how his pulmonary tree would be affected.
    ANSWER: Since asthma is an obstructive pulmonary process, during an acute the pulmonary tree is affected in several important ways: 1) airway narrowing via bronchospasm / bronchoconstriction, and 2) airway obstruction through pooling of tenacious secretions

10. Tom has an uncle, whose name is Henry. Henry was diagnosed with chronic bronchitis and emphysema ten years ago. On Henry's latest chest x-ray, it was noted that he had evidence of *cor pulmonale*. First briefly explain what cor pulmonale is. Second describe the significance of this pulmonary complication to Uncle Henry's long term health outcomes.
    ANSWERS: Answer #1) Cor pulmonale is right ventricular hypertrophy and dilation secondary to pulmonary disease. It is associated with increased pulmonary vascular resistance secondary to chronic hypoxemia. Answer #2) His cor pulmonale is a leading cause of death in COPD patients due to right heart failure.

SECTION SEVEN: ACUTE RESPIRATORY FAILURE

11. During his hospital stay, Tom develops acute respiratory failure. Briefly differentiate respiratory failure from respiratory insufficiency.
    ANSWER: The difference between respiratory insufficiency and failure is a matter of compensatory status. When a patient develops respiratory insufficiency, he/she is able to maintain relatively normal arterial blood gases due to intact compensatory mechanisms, particularly the heart. When a person develops respiratory failure, he/she is no longer to adequately compensate and ABGs become abnormal which , if left untreated, can lead to death.

12. In your own words, define acute (adult) respiratory distress syndrome (ARDS).
    TEXT ANSWER: "a distinct type of respiratory failure caused by diffuse injury to the alveolar-capillary membrane, resulting in noncardiogenic pulmonary edema"

13. Tom has been developing increasing symptoms of hypoxemia throughout the day. The physician orders oxygen therapy. If Tom has developed ARDS, the nurse would anticipate that his oxygen therapy would have what effect on his oxygenation status?

    ANSWER: Since the hallmark of ARDS is refractory hypoxemia, one would anticipate that administering oxygen to Tom will have no significant effect on improving his oxygenation. This is due to the presence of significant absolute shunt associated with ARDS.

14. Tom's latest PaO_2 on 100 % oxygen therapy is 58 mm Hg. According to Table 3-8, what can be said about his PaO_2?

    ANSWER: There are several important pieces of information that can be obtained from the table. First, his hypoxemia status would be considered moderate (< 60 mm Hg but > 40 mm Hg). Second, since he is receiving oxygen therapy, his 58 mm Hg PaO_2 would be considered "uncorrected hypoxemia".

SECTION EIGHT: RESPIRATORY ASSESSMENT

15. Briefly explain why the nurse should obtain a nutritional history from Tom.

    ANSWER: Assessing his nutritional status at admission may provide the health care team with important clues regarding his overall nutritional state. If he has an underlying malnutrition, particularly protein-calorie, his deficiency of protein can weaken his respiratory muscles as well as negatively affect his immune status.

16. The nurse should assess Tom for the three most common complaints associated with pulmonary disorders. These include:

    1. *dyspnea*
    2. *chest pain*
    3. *cough*
    4. *sputum and hemoptysis*

17. Tom is complaining of shortness of breath. The nurse charts that he is dyspneic. Dyspnea is a(n) ***subjective*** / objective (circle one) term. It is associated with increased ***work of breathing***.

18. Tom is complaining of chest pain. If his description of the pain he is experiencing is typical of pleuritic pain, you would expect to describe in as:

    ANSWER: Pleuritic pain is typically described as being sharp and knife-like. Tom may be able to point to it at a precise location. When asked to hold his breath, the pain is often reduced or absent.

19. Tom is coughing up secretions. In the absence of infection, Tom's secretions should have what appearance?

    ANSWER: thin, clear secretions

20. You are auscultating Tom's chest. When you place your stethoscope over the area of his pneumonia, you would probably hear what types of adventitious breath sounds?

    ANSWER: Crackles (rales) may be heard over the affected lung. Additionally, the nurse may hear bronchial (tubular) sounds over the same area (abnormal). If Tom has significant secretions, the nurse may hear rhonchi in the major airways. If the pneumonia causes an inflammation of his pleural membranes, a pleural rub may be auscultated. If, however, the affected lung tissue is consolidated, no breath sounds may be heard over that area due to lack of airflow.

SECTION NINE: RESPIRATORY CALCULATIONS

21. The ideal Alveolar Gas Equation is a method of measuring what respiratory related gas factor?
    ANSWER: P_{AO_2}, which is the partial pressure of alveolar oxygen. It is necessary to use this equation since P_{AO_2} cannot be measured directly.

22. Which of the respiratory calculations helps to estimate shunt? Which is considered <u>least</u> accurate?
    ANSWERS: #1) A-a gradient, a/A Ratio and PaO_2/FIO_2. #2) A-a gradient.

SECTION TEN: DEVELOPING A PULMONARY PLAN OF CARE

23. Assuming that the nurse needs to configure a plan of care using nursing diagnoses, which respiratory related nursing diagnosis focuses on the rate, rhythm and depth of breathing?
    ANSWER: Ineffective breathing pattern

24. You have just written the nursing diagnosis, Impaired gas exchange. What would be the most appropriate expected patient outcomes to measure this diagnosis?
    ANSWER: The two EPOS that most directly address this diagnosis are: " ABGs within normal limits for patient"; "usual mental status". Others include: absence of cyanosis, breathing unlabored, respiratory rate 12 to 20/minute, and no use of accessory respiratory muscles.

25. List at least 5 nursing interventions that would most likely be incorporated into Tom's plan of care if the nursing diagnosis: *Ineffective airway clearance* was written would include:
    ANSWER: Any of the following would be appropriate – Assess for ineffective airway clearance; assist in coughing and deep breathing every 1 to 2 hours; encourage fluids to 2 to 2.5 L per 24 hours; perform tracheal suctioning if necessary, monitor for effects of drug therapy; monitor for and treat acute pain; encourage self-care as tolerated; encourage activity and early ambulation, as tolerated

CONGRATULATIONS !!

YOU HAVE COMPLETED THIS STUDY GUIDE

Take Home Case
Module 4: Arterial Blood Gas Analysis

DIRECTIONS

In narrative form, complete the following questions or statements based on the Module reading assignment. To better comprehend this material, it is best to answer the items in your own words rather than copying answers from the text. you can evaluate what you actually understand and review what you do not.

READING ASSIGNMENT: *High Acuity Nursing, 2nd ed.* -- Module 4: Arterial Blood Gas Analysis
****

SITUATION: **Samantha W., 18 years old, is a student at a small local college. Two days ago, Samantha developed chills, a fever of 102.4, and a harsh cough. Today, Samantha began experiencing increasing shortness of breath and mental clouding. Her roommate took her to the campus infirmary. Following a preliminary evaluation at the infirmary, Samantha was transferred to the community hospital. She is diagnosed with a bacterial pneumonia.**

SECTION ONE:

1. Samantha is currently breathing room air which is composed of _____ percent of oxygen. This can be also represented as a partial pressure measurement. The partial pressure of room air is _____ mm Hg.

2. About _____ percent of the O_2 total content dissolves in the blood. What is the significance of this?

3. Diffusion of gas refers to the transfer of gas molecules from an area of _____ partial pressure to an area of _____ partial pressure.

4. When diffusion occurs at across the alveolar-capillary membranes, _____ (gas) moves into from the alveoli into the capillaries and _____ (gas) moves from the capillaries into the alveoli.

5. According to the oxyhemoglobin dissociation curve, what will happen to Samantha's hemoglobin saturation (SaO_2) if her PaO_2 falls below 60 mm Hg?

6. Samantha's high fever, if left unchecked, will have what effect on the oxyhemoglobin dissociation curve and to her oxygenation status?

SECTION TWO: ACID-BASE PHYSIOLOGY AND COMPENSATION

7. Differentiate volatile from nonvolatile acids. In what way are volatile acids of significance to Samantha?

8. What three mechanisms does Samantha's body use to maintain pH balance? In general, how does each work?

Mechanism	General Action

9. In your own words, describe each of the four levels of compensation:

Level of Compensation	Description
Uncompensated (Acute)	
Partially compensated	
Compensated (Chronic)	
Corrected	

SECTION THREE: NORMAL VALUES FOR ARTERIAL BLOOD GASES

10. In the space provided, differentiate the ABG components as directed:

Component	Acid-Base or Oxygenation Determinant	Normal Range	Description
pH			
$PaCO_2$			

Com-ponent	Acid-Base or Oxygenation Determinant	Normal Range	Description
HCO_3			
B E			
PaO_2			
SaO_2			
Hgb			

SECTION FOUR: RESPIRATORY ACID-BASE DISTURBANCE

11. What is the underlying cause of respiratory acidosis regardless of the etiology?

12. If Samantha should develop respiratory acidosis, which of the common causes would most likely be the etiology?

13. If Samantha develops respiratory alkalosis, it results from alveolar _____. What might precipitate this A-B disturbance early in her disease process?

14. If Samantha's current ABG shows partially compensated respiratory alkalosis, you would expect her bicarbonate level (HCO_3) to be: above normal range, below normal range, or within normal range? WHY?

15. If Samantha's ABG showed compensated respiratory acidosis, you would expect her $PaCO_2$ level to be: above normal range, below normal range, or within normal range? WHY?

SECTION FIVE: METABOLIC ACID-BASE DISTURBANCES

Samantha has been receiving several broad spectrum IV antibiotics.

16. If Samantha develops a primary metabolic acid-base disturbance, you would expect to see changes in which two metabolic components?

17. Examine the conditions that either increase hydrogen ion concentrations or decrease bicarbonate levels. Which of these most likely would apply to Samantha's situation?

18. If Samantha develops metabolic acidosis, what type of compensation would you expect?

19. If Samantha should develop severe vomiting, in what way can this disturb her acid-base balance?

20. Briefly explain why lactic acid levels are of interest in patients who are at risk for developing shock.

SECTION SIX: ARTERIAL BLOOD GAS INTERPRETATION

An Arterial Blood Gas Analysis exercise is provided at the end of the Case Studies/Exercise section *(These exercises are for interpretation practice only, they are not necessarily realistic ABG values)*

SECTION SEVEN: INTERPRETATION OF MIXED ACID-BASE DISORDERS

21. Write a brief explanation of the concept of "mixed acid-base disorders". How do they differ from a simple acid-base disorder?

22. The text explains that mixed disorders can have either a nullifying effect or an additive effect. What does this statement mean?

23. When reading ABG results, under what circumstances should you suspect that a mixed acid-base problem is present?

24. What are the three predictable blood gas relationships?

SECTION EIGHT: NONINVASIVE MONITORING OF GAS EXCHANGE

25. Samantha has pulse oximetry ordered. What does it measure?

26. What factors can alter the accuracy of Samantha's pulse oximetry?

27. Where can the pulse oximetry sensor be placed?

28. What is capnometry? What is its single value measurement?

29. Under what circumstances would capnometry most likely be considered for Samantha?

CONGRATULATIONS !! YOU HAVE COMPLETED THIS CASE

Take Home Case
Module 4: Arterial Blood Gas Analysis
Instructor Guide

DIRECTIONS

In narrative form, complete the following questions or statements based on the Module reading assignment. To better comprehend this material, it is best to answer the items in your own words rather than copying answers from the text. By do so, you can evaluate what you actually understand.

READING ASSIGNMENT: *High Acuity Nursing, 2nd ed.* -- Module 4: Arterial Blood Gas Analysis
****

SITUATION: Samantha W., 18 years old, is a student at a small local college. Two days ago, Samantha developed chills, f ever of 102.4, and a harsh cough. Today, Samantha began experiencing increasing shortness of breath and mental clouding. Her roommate took her to the campus infirmary. Following a preliminary evaluation at the infirmary, Samantha was transferred to the community hospital. She is diagnosed with a bacterial pneumonia.

SECTION ONE:

1. Samantha is currently breathing room air which is composed of _____*21*___ percent of oxygen. This can be also represented as a partial pressure measurement. The partial pressure of room air is _*158*___ mm Hg.

2. About _____ percent of the O_2 total content dissolves in the blood. What is the significance of this?
   ANSWERS: 3. When an ABG is drawn, the PaO_2 is actually measuring only the 3 % of dissolved oxygen in the circulation. Therefore, it can only indirectly reflect total oxygen content in the blood.

3. Diffusion of gas refers to the transfer of gas molecules from an area of _*high*___ partial pressure to an area of *low* partial pressure.

4. When diffusion occurs at across the alveolar-capillary membranes, ___*oxygen*___ (gas) moves into from the alveoli into the capillaries and ___*carbon dioxide*___ (gas) moves from the capillaries into the alveoli.

5. According to the oxyhemoglobin dissociation curve, what will happen to Samantha's hemoglobin saturation (SaO_2) if her PaO_2 falls below 60 mm Hg?
   ANSWER: At the lower part of the curve (≤ 60 mm Hg) a small decrease in PaO_2 will result in a large decrease in hemoglobin saturation (SaO_2). Assuming the V/Q relationship is normal, administering oxygen therapy should yield a rapid increase in SaO_2.

6. Samantha's high fever, if left unchecked, will have what effect on the oxyhemoglobin dissociation curve and to her oxygenation status?
   ANSWER: It will shift the curve to the right, which inhibits the ability of oxygen to bind with hemoglobin. At the tissue level, it increases the ability of bound oxygen to be released to the tissues. This can lead to a supply and demand problem (less available bound O_2 for exchange, high demand and rapid transfer of bound O_2 to the tissues. Ultimately, Samantha is at risk for developing hypoxemia.

SECTION TWO: ACID-BASE PHYSIOLOGY AND COMPENSATION

7. Differentiate volatile from nonvolatile acids. In what way are volatile acids of significance to Samantha?
   ANSWER: Volatile acids convert to gas form to be excreted (e.g., carbonic acid) while nonvolatile acids must be excreted through the kidneys (e.g., lactic acid, ketones). If Samantha's lungs do not

ventilate adequately, carbonic acid levels will increase in the body, leading to respiratory acidosis. If the kidneys are not working adequately, nonvolatile acids will build up and metabolic acidosis will develop.

8. What three mechanisms does Samantha's body use to maintain pH balance? In general, how does each work?

Mechanism	General Action
Buffering	*Uses chemical reactions between acids and bases to maintain a neutral environment. The major reversible reaction is:* $H^+ + HCO_3 \leftrightarrow H_2CO_3 \leftrightarrow CO_2 + H_2O$
Respiratory Compensation	*Increases or decreases alveolar ventilation. Hyperventilation leads to $\downarrow CO_2$ levels (therefore $\downarrow H_2CO_3$) and $\uparrow$ pH. Hypoventilation leads to $\uparrow CO_2$ levels (therefore $\uparrow H_2CO_3$) and $\downarrow$ pH.*
Metabolic Compensation	*Compensates through rate of elimination or reabsorption of H^+ and HCO_3^- in the kidneys.*

9. In your own words, describe each of the four levels of compensation:

Level of Compensation	Description
Uncompensated (Acute)	*Text def.: The pH is abnormal because buffer and regulatory mechanisms have not begun to correct the imbalance. In these situations, the acid or base component is abnormal.*
Partially compensated	*Text def.: The pH is abnormal, but the body buffers and regulatory mechanisms have started to respond to the imbalance. In these situations, the acid and base components are abnormal.*
Compensated (Chronic)	*Text def.: The pH is within normal limits. The acid-base imbalance has been neutralized but not corrected. In this situation, the acid and base components are abnormal but balanced.*
Corrected	*The pH is within normal limits. All acid-base parameters have returned to normal ranges after a state of acid-base imbalance.*

SECTION THREE: NORMAL VALUES FOR ARTERIAL BLOOD GASES

10. In the space provided, differentiate the ABG components as directed:

Component	Acid-Base or Oxygenation Determinant	Normal Range	Description
pH	*A-B*	*7.35-7.45*	*Represents amount of free H+ available in blood.*
PaCO$_2$	*A-B*	*35-45 mm Hg*	*Represents respiratory component of ABG.*
HCO$_3$	*A-B*	*24-28 mEq/L*	*Represents renal or metabolic component of ABG.*
Base Excess	*A-B*	*± 2 mEq/L*	*Indirectly reflects bicarbonate concentration in body.*
PaO$_2$	*Oxygenation*	*75-100 mm Hg*	*Represents amount of dissolved O_2 in arterial blood not the total amount of O_2 available.*
SaO$_2$	*Oxygenation*	*95-100%*	*The measure of percentage of oxygen combined with hemoglobin compared to the total amount it could carry.*

Component	Acid-Base or Oxygenation Determinant	Normal Range	Description
Hemoglobin	*Oxygenation*	*13.5-17 g/dL (males)* *12-15 g/dL (females)*	*The major component of RBCs. Oxygen is carried on the heme portion*

SECTION FOUR: RESPIRATORY ACID-BASE DISTURBANCE

11. What is the underlying cause of respiratory acidosis regardless of the etiology?
    ANSWER: Regardless of what has precipitated it, respiratory acidosis is caused by alveolar hypoventilation.

12. If Samantha should develop respiratory acidosis, which of the common causes would most likely be the etiology?
    ANSWER: Her pneumonia will affect the small airways, altering diffusion. CO_2 will be retained, causing a decreased pH

13. If Samantha develops respiratory alkalosis, it results from alveolar __*hyperventilation*____. What might precipitate this A-B disturbance early in her disease process?
    ANSWER: Her fever and hypoxia will cause her to hyperventilate, blowing off CO_2. It is quite common in early pneumonia.

14. If Samantha's current ABG shows partially compensated respiratory alkalosis, you would expect her bicarbonate level (HCO_3) to be: above normal range, below normal range, or within normal range? WHY?
    ANSWER: below the normal range; because respiratory acid-base problems are compensated through metabolic mechanisms. The kidneys will increase excretion of bicarbonate to lower the pH.

15. If Samantha's ABG showed compensated respiratory acidosis, you would expect her $PaCO_2$ level to be: above normal range, below normal range, or within normal range? WHY?
    ANSWER: above normal range; while the pH is now normal, her acid-base problem has not been corrected. This means that her $PaCO_2$ is still abnormal but HCO_3 (and other buffers) have been retained in sufficient quantities to reestablish a normal pH.

SECTION FIVE: METABOLIC ACID-BASE DISTURBANCES

Samantha has been receiving several broad spectrum IV antibiotics.

16. If Samantha develops a primary metabolic acid-base disturbance, you would expect to see changes in which two metabolic components?
    ANSWER: HCO_3 and BE

17. Examine the conditions that either increase hydrogen ion concentrations or decrease bicarbonate levels. Which of these most likely would apply to Samantha's situation?
    ANSWER: Her antibiotic therapy may kill off her normal GI flora, causing severe diarrhea. Of the conditions noted in the Section 5 lists, diarrhea is the most likely source, creating an increased loss of bicarbonate and metabolic acidosis.

18. If Samantha develops metabolic acidosis, what type of compensation would you expect?
    ANSWER: The lungs will hyperventilate to increase the loss of CO_2. Therefore, $PaCO_2$ levels will decrease.

19. If Samantha should develop severe vomiting, in what way can this disturb her acid-base balance?
    ANSWER: It can cause a loss of gastric fluids which results in loss of acid. This can cause

metabolic alkalosis.

20. Briefly explain why lactic acid levels are of interest in patients who are at risk for developing shock.
    ANSWER: Shock is associated with cellular hypoxia, which drives lactic acid levels up rapidly. Levels often rise before the patient begins to decompensate, thus lactic acidosis may be indicative of impending shock. Use of lactic acid levels then can potentially improve patient outcomes if the patient is treated for shock effectively prior to decompensation.

SECTION SIX: ARTERIAL BLOOD GAS INTERPRETATION

[An ABG Analysis Exercise is provided at the end of the Case Studies/Exercise section]
(This exercise is for interpretation practice only, the examples are not necessarily realistic ABG values)

SECTION SEVEN: INTERPRETATION OF MIXED ACID-BASE DISORDERS

[Instructor, you may want to consider this section as optional reading. I included it because teachers struggle with this concept continuously.]

21. Write a brief explanation of the concept of "mixed acid-base disorders". How do they differ from a simple acid-base disorder?
    ANSWER: A mixed acid-base disorder is a complex problem in which there are several primary acid base disturbances present simultaneously, requiring a more complex compensatory response. A simple A-B disorder has only one primary acid-base disturbance with one secondary acid-base compensatory response.

22. The text explains that mixed disorders can have either a nullifying effect or an additive effect. What does this statement mean?
    ANSWER: The nullifying effect refers to the presence of two acid-base disturbances that rebalance the pH. (e.g., a metabolic alkalosis state that is present with a respiratory acidosis state). One pulls the pH up while the other pulls it down. This tends to minimize the pH derangement. The additive effect refers to the presence of several disturbances that are both either acidosis or alkalosis (e.g., primary respiratory acidosis and primary metabolic acidosis), the pH derangement will be worse than if either existed alone.

23. When reading ABG results, under what circumstances should you suspect that a mixed acid-base problem is present?
    ANSWER: The clinician should suspect a mixed problem when either the $PaCO_2$ or the HCO_3 is: 1) in a direction opposite its predicted direction, or 2) not close to the predicted value, during normal compensatory activity.

24. What are the three predictable blood gas relationships?
    ANSWER: pH to HCO_3; pH to $PaCO_2$; and $PaCO_2$ to HCO_3 relationships.

SECTION EIGHT: NONINVASIVE MONITORING OF GAS EXCHANGE

25. Samantha has pulse oximetry ordered. What does it measure?
    ANSWER: It measures arterial capillary hemoglobin saturation by determining oxyhemoglobin saturation.

26. What factors can alter the accuracy of Samantha's pulse oximetry?
    ANSWER: Technical factors, such as bright light sources in environment, improperly placed sensors, and misinterpreted body movements. Physiologic factors, such as hemoglobin, acid-base imbalance, and peripheral vasoconstriction.

27. Where can the pulse oximetry sensor be placed?
    ANSWER: finger, nose, and ear are most common locations

28. What is capnometry? What is its single value measurement?

 ANSWER: Capnometry is the noninvasive measurement of carbon dioxide concentration in expired gas; $PETCO_2$.

29. Under what circumstances would capnometry most likely be considered for Samantha?

 ANSWER: If she is at risk for significant alterations in ventilatory status, it can provide an early warning of impending, either hypoventilation or hyperventilation related problems.

Take Home Case
Module 5: Mechanical Ventilation

DIRECTIONS:
      In narrative form, complete the following questions or statements based on the Module reading assignment. To better comprehend the material, it is best to answer the items in your own words rather than copying answers from the text. You can evaluate what you actually understand and review what you do not.

READING ASSIGNMENT: *High Acuity Nursing, 2nd ed.* -- Module 5: Mechanical Ventilation
****

> SITUATION: *Phyllis T. is a 76 year old retired college teacher who was admitted to the hospital with a diagnosis of pneumonia. Subsequent to her admission, she required mechanical ventilation to treat her acute respiratory failure.*

SECTION ONE: VENTILATOR VS RESPIRATOR
1.   The machine that is assisting Phyllis in breathing is a mechanical ventilator, not a respirator. Briefly explain the difference between ventilation and respiration.

SECTION TWO: DETERMINING THE NEED FOR VENTILATORY SUPPORT

2.   Before Phyllis received mechanical ventilation support, it was determined that she met certain criteria. In the space provided, write a brief description of each criteria:

Criteria	Objective Criteria	Brief Description
Acute Ventilatory Failure (AVF)		
Hypoxemia		
Pulmonary Mechanics		

SECTION THREE: REQUIRED EQUIPMENT FOR MECHANICAL VENTILATION

3.   You are the nurse who is responsible for setting up the equipment needed to intubate Phyllis. List all of the items that should be available to actually intubate her:

4.   In addition to the intubation equipment, what other supportive equipment is needed to support her respiratory status?

5.   Is it likely that they would do a tracheostomy on Phyllis initially? Why or why not?

6.   In your own words, briefly describe how to secure an endotracheal tube in place directly following intubation:

SECTION FOUR: TYPES OF MECHANICAL VENTILATORS

6.   Briefly explain the difference between a negative pressure ventilator and positive pressure ventilators:

7.   Why do you think that high acuity patients, such as Phyllis, are placed on positive pressure ventilators rather than negative pressure ventilators?

8.   A Volume-Cycled Ventilator delivers a preset _____ of gas to the lungs. A Time-Cycled Ventilator controls _____ allowed for inspiration.

SECTION FIVE: COMMONLY MONITORED VENTILATOR SETTINGS

9. Match the following ventilator settings with the correct facts that apply to each of them. (NOTE: there may be more than one for each item)

Setting		*Fact*
_____ Tidal Volume	A.	measurement of the amount of pressure required to deliver a volume of air
_____ FiO$_2$	B.	room air is 0.21
_____ Assist / Control	C.	provides alveoli with a constant amount of positive pressure at the end of each expiration; requires mechanical ventilation
_____ IMV	D.	the amount of air that moves in and out of the lungs in one normal breath
_____ Rate	E.	normal range is 7 to 9 mL/kg
_____ PEEP	F.	a combined ventilation mode that is patient sensitive. The patient is able to initiate inhalation, with a time back-up mechanism
_____ CPAP	G.	part of the minute ventilation equation
_____ PSV	H.	a ventilation mode that allows the patient to spontaneously breathe through the ventilator circuit
_____ PIP	I.	refers to fraction of inspired oxygen. It is expressed as a decimal
	J.	provides positive pressure to the alveoli during the inhalation phase to augment the tidal volume
	K.	delivers a continuous flow of positive pressure such that the airway pressure never drops to zero; does not require mechanical ventilation

10. Briefly explain the controversy regarding high vs. low tidal volumes during mechanical ventilation:

11. Phyllis's ventilator will have a variety of alarms activated. In the space provided, list the common causes of a low pressure alarm and high pressure alarms:

Low Pressure Alarms

High Pressure Alarms

SECTION SIX: NONINVASIVE ALTERNATIVES TO MECHANICAL VENTILATION

12. What type of patient problems might be treated using NIPPV?

13. Describe the masks used for noninvasive breathing support, including how they are kept in place:

14. List at least five beneficial effects of NIPPV:

15. For the various complications associated with NIPPV noted in the left column, list the usual cause and appropriate treatment in the two right columns:

Complication	Usual Cause	Treatment
Conjunctivitis		
Gastric distention		
Nasal problems		
Skin irritation		
Hypoventilation Syndrome		

SECTION SEVEN: MAJOR COMPLICATIONS OF MECHANICAL VENTILATION

16. Briefly describe what effects positive pressure ventilation will have on Phyllis's:

Cardiovascular system:

Pulmonary status:

Neurovascular status:

Renal status:

Gastrointestinal status:

18. Complete the following sentences that summarize concepts regarding major complications of mechanical ventilation that Phyllis will need to be closely monitored for:

Because her cardiac output will be less, the nurse will closely monitor her for development of decreased _____, increased _____, and development of cardiac _____.

The nurse will monitor Phyllis's pulmonary status for signs of barotrauma, which would include sudden onset of _____, _____, _____, or _____.

If Phyllis requires high concentrations of oxygen for more than 48 hours, she is at risk for developing _____.

The presence of the ET tube places Phyllis at high risk for pulmonary infection. If infection is suspected, two tests/procedures that will probably be ordered including: _____ and _____.

To prevent gastrointestinal complications, Phyllis' physicians may order histamine (H2) antagonists to increase / decrease her gastric pH.

SECTION EIGHT: ARTIFICIAL AIRWAY COMPLICATIONS

18. Briefly describe how artificial airways can cause nasal damage:

19. How can pressure from the artificial airway cuff damage Phyllis's trachea?

Cuff trauma can be minimized by maintaining a cuff pressure of between ____ and ____ mm Hg.

SECTION NINE: CARE OF THE PATIENT REQUIRING MECHANICAL VENTILATION

20. Ineffective airway clearance is a priority nursing diagnosis in managing the mechanically ventilated patient. Briefly explain why this is particular problem in this patient population.

21. True / False (circle one) The mechanically ventilated patient should be suctioned every one to two hours throughout the 24 hour period.

22. If Phyllis is placed on PEEP, what negative effects can suctioning have on her status? How can these problems be reduced?

23. What three nursing interventions will decrease pooling of secretions in mechanically ventilated patients?

24. If the ventilator rate and/or tidal volume are set too high, Phyllis will develop alveolar _____, which will cause this acid-base imbalance: _____. If the ventilator rate and/or tidal volume are set too low, Phyllis will develop alveolar _____, which will cause this acid-base imbalance: _____.

25. Name three nursing interventions that will help protect Phyllis's airway:

26. Briefly explain why Phyllis's nutritional state will need to be evaluated and closely monitored throughout her hospitalization.

27. List three common psychosocial problems associated with patients requiring mechanical ventilation:

SECTION TEN: WEANING THE PATIENT FROM THE MECHANICAL VENTILATOR

28. What is the purpose of performing a "Simple Screening" for determination of readiness to wean?

29. During a comprehensive patient screening for determination of readiness to wean, why do the criteria involve evaluation of multiple systems?

30. The term "manual weaning" refers to:

31. During manual weaning, what is the role of the nurse?

32. The term "ventilator weaning" refers to:

32. Match the descriptions in the right column to the correct type of ventilator weaning mode in the left column (There can be more than one correct match):

Weaning Mode	*Description*
_____ IMV/SIMV	A. Provides good control of $PaCO_2$
_____ PSV	B. A disadvantage is that all breaths are spontaneous
_____ MMV	C. The frequency of mandatory breaths is slowly decreased
	D. Supports tidal volume, decreasing work of breathing
	E. The most common type of ventilator weaning

34. When Phyllis is completely weaned, she will need to be extubated. What type of equipment will need to be present for use directly following extubation?

35. What types of nursing interventions can the nurse anticipate post extubation?

CONGRATULATIONS!!
YOU HAVE COMPLETED THIS THC

Take Home Case
Module 5: Mechanical Ventilation
Instructor Guide

READING ASSIGNMENT: *High Acuity Nursing, 2nd ed.* -- Module 5: Mechanical Ventilation
****

> *SITUATION: Phyllis T. is a 76 year old retired college teacher who was admitted to the hospital with a diagnosis of pneumonia. Subsequent to her admission, she required mechanical ventilation to treat her acute respiratory failure.*

SECTION ONE: VENTILATOR VS RESPIRATOR

1. The machine that is assisting Phyllis in breathing is a mechanical ventilator, not a respirator. Briefly explain the difference between ventilation and respiration:
   The term Ventilation refers to the gross movement of air in and out of the lungs. The term respiration refers to the exchange of oxygen and carbon dioxide across a semi-permeable membrane.

SECTION TWO: DETERMINING THE NEED FOR VENTILATORY SUPPORT

2. Before Phyllis received mechanical ventilation support, it was determined that she met certain criteria. In the space provided, write a brief description of each criteria:

Criteria	Objective Criteria	Brief Description
Acute Ventilatory Failure (AVF)	*$PaCO_2 > 50$ mm Hg and pH < 7.30*	*The inability of the lungs to maintain adequate alveolar ventilation. Diagnosed on basis of the a-b imbalance it creates. Clinically, it refers to acute respiratory acidosis.*
Hypoxemia	*PaO_2 of < 50 mm Hg*	*The most common cause is a low V/Q ratio. Examples of conditions that cause a low V/Q ratio include: asthma, pneumonia, COPD, and atelectasis.* *Low V/Q ratio is associated with right-to-left shunt*
Pulmonary Mechanics	*RR (f) = > 35/minute* *VC = < 15 mL/kg* *NIF = < -20 cm/H_2O* *VE = > 10 L/minute*	*Pulmonary tests that provide the clinician with information about respiratory muscle strength and airflow.*

SECTION THREE: REQUIRED EQUIPMENT FOR MECHANICAL VENTILATION

3. You are the nurse who is responsible for setting up the equipment needed to intubate Phyllis. List all of the items that should be available to actually intubate her:
   Endotracheal tube; Stylet; topical anesthetic; laryngoscope handle with blade attached; Magill forceps; Yankauers pharyngeal suction tip; syringe for cuff inflation; water-soluble lubricant; adhesive tape

4. In addition to the intubation equipment, what other supportive equipment is needed to support her respiratory status?
   Supportive equipment includes: two oxygen sources (one for vent; one for ambu bag); suction equipment and sterile suction catheters; cuff manometer to check cuff pressure; manual resuscitation bag;

SECTION FOUR: TYPES OF MECHANICAL VENTILATORS

5. Is it likely that a tracheostomy would be performed on Phyllis initially? Why or why not?

No; unless she has an obstruction in the upper airway, a tracheostomy is generally considered too invasive of a procedure, too time consuming and unnecessary, initially.

6. In your own words, briefly describe why it is crucial to secure an endotracheal tube in place directly following intubation:
    An unstable ET tube can be easily dislodged or completely pulled out by accident. This can lead to rapid respiratory compromise. Reintubation may be more difficult and traumatic than the initial procedure.

7. Briefly explain the difference between a negative pressure ventilator and positive pressure ventilator:
    Negative pressure ventilators apply negative pressure externally. The patient's thorax (or body) is sealed in an airtight container and air pressure in the container is reduced to below atmospheric at regular intervals causing the thoracic cage to lift. These ventilators do not require artificial airways and maintain fairly normal breathing mechanics.

    Positive pressure ventilators drive gases into the lungs through the ventilator's circuitry, which is attached to an artificial airway.

8. A Volume-Cycled Ventilator delivers a preset _*Volume*_ of gas to the lungs. A Time-Cycled Ventilator controls __*the time*__ allowed for inspiration.

SECTION FIVE: COMMONLY MONITORED VENTILATOR SETTINGS

9. Match the following ventilator settings with the correct facts that apply to each of them. (NOTE: there may be more than one for each item)

Setting		*Fact*
_D,E,G_ Tidal Volume	A.	measurement of the amount of pressure required to deliver a volume of air
_B,I_ FiO$_2$	B.	room air is 0.21
_F_ Assist / Control	C.	provides alveoli with a constant amount of positive pressure at the end of each expiration; requires mechanical ventilation
_H_ IMV	D.	the amount of air that moves in and out of the lungs in one normal breath
_G_ Rate	E.	normal range is 7 to 9 mL/kg
_C_ PEEP	F.	a combined ventilation mode that is patient sensitive. The patient is able to initiate inhalation, with a time back-up mechanism
_K_ CPAP	G.	part of the minute ventilation equation
_J_ PSV	H.	a ventilation mode that allows the patient to spontaneously breathe through the ventilator circuit
_A_ PIP	I.	refers to fraction of inspired oxygen. It is expressed as a decimal
	J.	provides positive pressure to the alveoli during the inhalation phase to augment the tidal volume
	K.	delivers a continuous flow of positive pressure such that the airway pressure never drops to zero; does not require mechanical ventilator

10. Briefly explain the controversy regarding high-volume vs. low volume tidal volumes during mechanical ventilation:
    Standard practice has been high tidal volumes for many years, to open up more alveoli, thus enhancing oxygenation and ventilation. However, high pressures on alveoli causes lung damage. There is growing interest in reducing tidal volumes and adding sighs, to decrease lung injury risks.

11. Phyllis's ventilator will have a variety of alarms activated. In the space provided, list the common causes of a low pressure alarm and high pressure alarms:

Low Pressure Alarms
> *Indicates loss of tidal volume or leak in system (e.g., leaking or inadequately filled cuff, tubing disconnection)*

High Pressure Alarms
> *Anything that increases airway resistance (e.g., coughing, biting tube, secretions in airway, water in tubing, deteriorating pulmonary condition (increasing compliance)*

SECTION SIX: NONINVASIVE ALTERNATIVES TO MECHANICAL VENTILATION

12. What type of patient problems might be treated using NIPPV?
> *Patients with one of three types of disorders: <u>neuromuscular</u>, such as spinal cord injury, muscular dystrophy, or hypoventilation syndrome; <u>restrictive</u>, such as severe obesity and chest wall restriction; or <u>obstructive</u>, such as severe cystic fibrosis and COPD.*

13. Describe the masks used for noninvasive breathing support, including how they are kept in place:
> *The mask covers either the mouth and the nose (oronasal) or just the nose(nasal). The mask is kept in place by straps that when secured properly should minimize or eliminate air leakage.*

14. List at least five beneficial effects of NIPPV:
> *They: avoid need for/eliminate use of tracheostomy, decrease inspiratory muscle energy expenditure, decrease incidence of nocturnal desaturation, improve daytime blood gases, increase daytime lung volumes, increase respiratory muscle strength and endurance, improve nocturnal gas exchange, improve daytime functioning and activity level, decease incidence of daytime headache, decrease daytime insomnia or somnolence, improve intellectual capacity.*

15. For the various complications associated with NIPPV noted in the left column, list the usual cause and appropriate treatment in the two right columns:

Complication	*Usual Cause*	*Treatment*
Conjunctivitis	*Air leaking out from mask around bridge of nose and blowing into eyes*	*May or may not be easy to correct. Mask needs to be resecured for better fit. May require new mask. Masks require changing at least every 3 months.*
Gastric distention	*Air swallowing*	*Sleep in lateral position; use abdominal strap. Symptoms may eventually decrease.*
Nasal problems	*Drying of nasal membranes with air*	*Use humidification (in-line, nasal sprays, room).*
Skin irritation	*Irritation from mask straps*	*Daily cleaning of mask and straps*
Hypoventilation Syndrome	*Inadequate seal to attain needed pressure; inadequate air flow*	*Improve mask seal; adjust air flow, if possible.*

SECTION SEVEN: MAJOR COMPLICATIONS OF MECHANICAL VENTILATION

16. Briefly describe what effects positive pressure ventilation will have on Phyllis':

Cardiovascular system:
> *Increased CVP, decreased C.O., decreased right heart preload, decreased right heart stroke volume. It also squeezes the heart during the inspiratory phase.*

Pulmonary status:
> *Gas will follow the path of least resistance -- therefore, gas will flow more to nondependent lung areas and large airways. Alters the relationship between ventilation and perfusion.*

Neurovascular status:
> *Increases intracranial pressure, and decreases cerebral perfusion pressure*

Renal status:
> *Decreases urinary output through redistribution of blood flow*

Gastrointestinal status:
Decreases blood flow to intestinal viscera -- resulting tissue ischemia increases risk for gastric ulcer formation and GI bleeding.

17. Complete the following sentences that summarize major concepts regarding major complications of mechanical ventilation that Phyllis will need to be closely monitored for:

Because her cardiac output will be less, the nurse will closely monitor her for development of decreased __*blood pressure*_, increased _*pulse*_, and development of cardiac _*arrhythmias*_.

The nurse will monitor Phyllis' pulmonary status for signs of barotrauma, which would include sudden onset of _*agitation and cough assoc. with high pressure alarm*__, __*deteriorating BP and ABG*__, __*diminished or absent breath sounds*___, or __*subcutaneous emphysema*__.

If Phyllis requires high concentrations of oxygen for more than 48 hours, she is at risk for developing _*oxygen toxicity*__.

The presence of the ET tube places Phyllis at high risk for pulmonary infection. If infection is suspected, two tests/procedures that will probably be ordered include: __*chest x-ray*__ and __*sputum culture*__.

To prevent gastrointestinal complications, Phyllis' physicians may order histamine (H2) antagonists to *increase* her gastric pH.

SECTION EIGHT: ARTIFICIAL AIRWAY COMPLICATIONS

18. Briefly describe how artificial airways can cause nasal damage:
Insertion can traumatize the delicate nasal mucous membranes during passing of tube. Tissue ischemia or necrosis of the nares can develop due to high pressure of tube pressing against the internal nasal wall.

19. How can pressure from the artificial airway cuff damage Phyllis's trachea?
When cuff pressure exceeds the arterial capillary pressure in the trachea it compresses the capillaries, restricting flow of oxygen to the local tissues. In time, tissue ischemia develops and eventually tissue necrosis develops.

Cuff trauma can be minimized by maintaining a cuff pressure of between _20_ and _25_ mm Hg. (*or 27-34 cm H$_2$O*)

SECTION NINE: CARE OF THE PATIENT REQUIRING MECHANICAL VENTILATION

20. Ineffective airway clearance is a priority nursing diagnosis in managing the mechanically ventilated patient. Briefly explain why this is particular problem in this patient population:
The patient requiring mechanical ventilation has difficulty clearing secretions for a variety of reasons. If the patient has an ET tube, the length and lumen size of the tube prevents secretions from being coughed up, thus causing pooling of secretions in the lungs. The presence of excessive secretions often requires suctioning every one to two hours or even less. If the patient is dehydrated, secretions become thick and difficult to mobilize for removal. In a patient with a tracheostomy, respiratory muscle weakness or fatigue often significantly weakens the cough effort, thereby decreasing airway clearance. The closed mechanical ventilation breathing circuit keeps secretions within the circuit unless they are removed.

21. True / *False* (circle one) The mechanically ventilated patient should be suctioned every one to two hours throughout the 24 hour period.

22. If Phyllis is placed on PEEP, what negative effects can suctioning have on her status? How can these problems be reduced?

    It can precipitate oxygen desaturation and hemodynamic instability. Problems can be reduced by using some form of closed suction or open suction with a PEEP valve on the manual resuscitation (ambu) bag.

23. What three nursing interventions will decrease pooling of secretions in mechanically ventilated patients?

    Proper suctioning, liquefying secretions, turning every 1 to 2 hours

24. If the ventilator rate and/or tidal volume are set too high, Phyllis will develop alveolar _hyperventilation__, which will cause this acid-base imbalance: __*respiratory alkalosis*___. If the ventilator rate and/or tidal volume are set too low, Phyllis will develop alveolar __*hypoventilation*____, which will cause this acid-base imbalance: ___*respiratory acidosis*___.

25. Name three nursing interventions that will help protect Phyllis's airway:

    1) maintain sufficient slack on ventilator tubing to minimize tension on the airway during moving, 2) disconnect her from the vent. and manually ventilate during transfer into and out of bed, and 3) adequately secure the airway through correct taping or stabilizing device.

26. Briefly explain why Phyllis's nutritional state will need to be evaluated and closely monitored throughout her hospitalization:

    A malnourished state can significantly inhibit healing, increase her risk for further infection and weaken her respiratory muscles, making weaning from the ventilator a more difficult task and prolonging her hospitalization.

27. List three common psychosocial problems associated with patients requiring mechanical ventilation:

    1) anxiety; 2) sleep pattern disturbance, 3) impaired verbal communication.

SECTION TEN: WEANING THE PATIENT FROM THE MECHANICAL VENTILATOR

28. What is the purpose of performing a "Simple Screening" for determination of readiness to wean?

    Objective criteria can be used to guide practice The simple screening procedures are relatively simple to perform and bear little, if any, cost. The clinician can rapidly screen Phyllis for risk factors associated with failure to wean. In more complex situations, a more comprehensive set of criteria will be employed.

29. During a comprehensive patient screening for determination of readiness to wean, why do the criteria involve evaluation of multiple systems?

    Positive pressure ventilation negatively effects multiple body systems. In addition, patients requiring mechanical ventilation often have multisystem dysfunction based on the complex nature of their underlying acute and/or chronic disease. In weaning the complex patient, a significant dysfunction of one body system can diminish chances for successful weaning and/or alter weaning procedures.

30. The term "manual weaning" refers to:

    Intermittent removal of the patient from the ventilator on a schedule of increasing periods of time. While off of the ventilator, the patient receives humidified oxygen, usually through a T-piece.

31. During manual weaning, what is the role of the nurse?

    The nurse acts as a coach and monitor. Coaching involves calm reassurance and encouraging correct breathing rate and depth. Manual weaning is time intensive for the nurse who must closely monitor the patient for signs of weaning intolerance.

32. The term "ventilator weaning" refers to:
    Weaning the patient while he or she remains on the ventilator. It involves slow withdrawal of support.

33. Match the descriptions in the right column to the correct type of ventilator weaning mode in the left column (There can be more than one correct match):

Weaning Mode	*Description*
_E,C_ IMV/SIMV	A. Provides good control of $PaCO_2$
_B,D_ PSV	B. A disadvantage is that all breaths are spontaneous
_A__ MMV	C. The frequency of mandatory breaths is slowly decreased
	D. Supports tidal volume, decreasing work of breathing
	E. The most common type of ventilator weaning

34. When Phyllis is completely weaned, she will need to be extubated. What type of equipment will need be present for use directly following extubation?
    A cool humidified oxygen set up and suctioning equipment.

35. What types of nursing interventions can the nurse anticipate post extubation?
    The nurse will need to conduct excellent pulmonary hygiene: coughing and deep breathing and incentive spirometry. In addition, the ordered humidified oxygen needs to be maintained.

Case Study
The Case of Pearl M

You are the nurse assigned to 81 year old Pearl M., a transfer patient who is coming from the neurosurgical ICU. You have just been informed that Pearl has arrived and placed in her bed.

Recent History

Approximately four weeks ago, Pearl was an unrestrained passenger in an automobile accident in which the passenger side of the car was hit by another vehicle. She sustained facial lacerations, multiple fractures, including her right first rib and superior pelvic ramus. A right eye dehiscence with iris prolapse and a right pneumothorax were also diagnosed.

Past History

Pearl comes from a rural Tennessee setting. She has never been hospitalized previous to this admission. She has no history of asthma, coronary artery disease, diabetes mellitus or other chronic conditions. She has never smoked and denies use of alcohol. Her chart indicates that she had a mild case of pneumonia during the previous winter. One year ago she had bilateral cataract surgery with lens replacements. She takes no medication at home. She has four living children.

The Initial Appraisal

Upon walking into her room for the first time you quickly note the following:

General appearance: Pearl is an elderly Caucasian female. She has thick gray hair, a wrinkled face with her skin hanging loosely. Her lips are pink. She is wearing glasses which have tape covering the right lens. You note that a tracheostomy tube is in place with a velcro band securing it.

Signs of distress: You note that Pearl's breathing appears rapid. Her left eye is darting around the room and she has a worried look on her face. When you speak to her she makes good eye contact and begins to rapidly mouth sentences to you, although she is unable to vocalize.

Other: Pearl has an IV of 5% Dextrose and 0.45 Normal Saline infusing through a peripheral line in her left hand. Her tracheostomy dressing is noted to have greenish secretions on it.

Systematic Bedside Assessment

Head and Neck

Pearl is oriented to person, place and year. Her Glasgow Coma Scale is 11-T. She follows you with her left eye as you move around the bed. Her left eye reacts to light briskly and is 2.0 mm is size. Her right eye is nonreactive to light and is 4.0 mm in size. Her mucous membranes are pale-pink and somewhat dry. A small bore enteric tube is in place in her left nostril and is secured to her left cheek. No nasal abrasion is noted. No jugular vein distention is noted. She has a #8 Shiley Tracheostomy tube. You noted that she has a significant amount of white frothy secretions present which requires immediate suctioning. She is receiving oxygen of 30% per tracheostomy collar. You have difficulty understanding her communication attempts due to her rapid mouthing of words in full sentences. Several old lacerations are noted on her face which appear to be healing well. She is unable to tolerate a diet, as swallowing precipitates severe coughing episodes.

Chest

Pulmonary status: Rhonchi are heard throughout her lung fields. Left lung field expiratory wheeze is noted and crackles (rales) are heard in her bases, bilaterally. Her respiratory rate is currently 24/minute. She has had episodes in the ICU in which her respiratory rate increased to 56 per minute. The ICU nurses attributed the anxiety episodes to severe anxiety. Her breathing is moderately labored and quite shallow. You note that she is using her accessory muscles. Tactile fremitus is felt over her left upper field.

Cardiac status: S_1 and S_2 are auscultated. No murmur is noted. Her apical rate is regular at 100/minute.

Abdomen

Bowel sounds are auscultated in all four quadrants, normoactive. She denies tenderness. Her abdomen is distended and tight in the lower quadrants which prove to be tympanic on percussion. Her enteric feeding tube is checked for placement. Placement is verified. *Pulmocare*™ is infusing through the tube via a pump at 75mL/Hr. No trauma or skin breakdown is noted on her abdomen.

Pelvis

A contusion is noted over the right ramus, approximately 10 mm in diameter. Her perineal area is erythemic with a small patches of white "cottage cheese-like" discharge present. Pearl is complaining of severe perineal burning. She is voiding per bedpan. Her urine is amber colored and slightly cloudy, with a distinct odor. She has no bladder distention.

Extremities:

+3 peripheral pulses are assessed. Her capillary refill is less than three seconds. Nail beds are pale-pink. Slight edema is noted and her skin turgor is unremarkable. Her bilateral grips are equal. Her skin is warm and dry. Her skin hangs loosely from her frame.

Posterior:

Skin is warm and moist. No signs of edema or skin breakdown are noted. Several reddened areas are noted over the mid-back. Posterior lung field auscultation is performed and crackles and rhonchi are noted throughout the posterior fields, louder than the anterior assessment.

Vital Signs:

Currently: BP = 140/88; P = 102, regular; R = 28/minute, somewhat labored; T = 98.8 (o).
Her ranges over the past 48 hours:
$$BP = \frac{138 - 150}{88 - 90}, \quad P = 100 - 120/minute, \quad R = 20 - 30/minute, \quad T = 97.8 (o) - 99.2 (o)$$

Psychosocial Assessment:

This is her first hospitalization. Her daughter works in this hospital and can visit regularly. She appears to become frustrated with her inability to communicate satisfactorily and is unable to write notes very well. Over the past several days, she has had several more episodes of severe agitation, with accompanying significant BP and R elevations.

Significant Labs and Other Tests:

Serum:

WBC with differential: WBC = 14.2, Segs = 9500, Bands = 3100, Lymphs = 1000.
RBC: 4.14
Glucose = 176
BUN = 22, UN/Creatinine = 31
Electrolytes: Within normal ranges except for: Phosphorus = 2.3

Urine:

Urine culture and sensitivity is pending. Routine urinalysis: pH = 8.5, Protein = 1+

Stool:

Specimen is pending for possible clostridium difficile isolation. The chart indicates that Pearl had several bouts of severe diarrhea while in the ICU.

Portable Chest X-ray:

Patchy densities observed in lungs bilaterally with large right pleural effusion and left lower lobe atelectasis.

Intake and Output :

Last 24 hours: I = 2217 mL and O = 1255 mL
Last 48 hours: I = 2871 mL and O = 2170 mL.

Other Data
Weight:
Admission = 112 pounds. Last week = 105 pounds.   Most Current = 117.5 pounds

Arterial Blood Gases:
Prior to original intubation, on 100% oxygen per mask:

pH = 7.36, PCO_2 = 32, PO_2 = 64, HCO_3 = 26, SaO_2 = 77%.

Respirations at that time: Rate = 42/minute, labored and shallow.

1 hour after intubation/mechanical ventilation, on 50% oxygen:

pH = 7.36, PCO_2 =36, PO_2 =100, HCO_3 = 25, SaO_2 = 96%.

Respirations at that time: On assist/control mode at 14/minute. She was initiating respirations at 22-24 breaths per minute. Tidal volume was set at 750 cc.

1 hr prior to transfer from floor to the Intermediate Care Unit, on 30% oxygen:

pH = 7.32, PCO_2 = 52, PO_2 = 78, HCO_3 = 30, SaO_2 = 80%.

Respirations at this time were: rate = 38/min., very shallow and labored. Rhonchi heard throughout fields. Suctioning for large amounts of thin frothy white secretions.

Physician Orders:
Vital signs every 4 hours.
Up in chair TID.
Suction every 20 - 40 minutes.
Portable chest x-ray.
Oxygen @ 30% per tracheostomy collar.
Full liquid diet. Pulmocare @ 75 cc/hr. Strict I & O.
Urine for UA and C & S.
Call H.O. (House Officer) for T > 101(o).
Maintain patch over right eye unless wearing patched glasses.

Medications:
Neutro-Phos Cap. 1 TID
Cimetidine Liquid 300 mg PO Q 6 hours.
Mylanta 30 cc PO PRN
Nystatin Liquid 300 mg PO Q 6 hours
Nystatin Cream to perineal area PRN Q 4 hours.
Nitroglycerin Ointment 1-inch to anterior chest wall Q 8 hours.
Tylenol 650 mg PO PRN Q 4 hours.

Miscellaneous Data:

Her ICU stay was complicated by pneumonia. Two days after admission, she developed respiratory distress, requiring mechanical ventilation for 21 days for repeated problems with oxygenation and ventilation. On Day 4 she required a thoracentesis resulting in the withdrawal of 700 ml of serosanguinous fluid. On Day 10, she extubated herself, not requiring reintubation until the next day. On Day 13, she received a percutaneous tracheostomy.

 Two days after she was transferred to your floor, the physician's ordered that she be transferred to the Intermediate Care Unit for closer monitoring of her respiratory status and more frequent suctioning (she has been requiring suctioning every 15 - 30 minutes).

The Case of Pearl M.: Study Guide

1. After you have read the Case Scenario of Pearl M., go through the data that is available on Pearl and underline or highlight all abnormal or suspicious data, beginning with the Recent History.

2. Once you have marked all abnormal/suspicious data, examine the data found in the **Initial Appraisal**. What abnormal or suspicious data did you find there? What general problem areas do these data fall into (e.g., cardiovascular, nutritional, psychosocial, etc.)?

3. Go to the clustering grid (Item #6). Document the general problem areas that you have already identified in the Initial Appraisal and the corresponding data that support it.

4. Based on your findings in 2, which part of your systematic bedside assessment should you perform first?

5. Now move on to Pearl's **Systematic Bedside Assessment, and Significant Labs and Other Tests** Examine the assessment data that you have selected as abnormal or suspicious. Enter these new findings onto the clustering grid.

> **NOTE**: You should be clustering data according to *critical cues*. All nursing diagnoses (and medical diagnoses) have critical cues that consist of a few pieces of data that strongly indicate the presence of a particular problem, disorder, or disease. For example, the nursing diagnosis, *fluid volume excess* is supported by criteria such as: Intake > Output, edema, + JVD, and adventitious breath sounds (crackles). The medical diagnosis *acute renal failure* is supported by abnormally high BUN and Creatinine serum levels, and clinical manifestations of fluid excess. Your data can fit into more than one data cluster – many will. *Suggestion*: begin with the most obvious and/or critical of the data cues and then add additional supportive data. Each data cluster should contain at least three pieces of data.]

6. **Data Clustering:** Data clusters do not have to be placed in any order of priorities. Rather, it is suggested that you list them in order of how you discover them. Numbers are provided to help you identify clusters.

DATA CLUSTERING GRID		
	Abnormal/Suspicious Data	*Problem Area*
1		
	Additional Data Needed:	
2		
	Additional Data Needed:	
3		
	Additional Data Needed:	

	DATA CLUSTERING GRID	
	Abnormal/Suspicious Data	Problem Area
4		
	Additional Data Needed:	
5		
	Additional Data Needed:	
6		
	Additional Data Needed:	
7		
	Additional Data Needed:	
8		
	Additional Data Needed:	

7. Once you have accounted for all of your abnormal / suspicious data through clustering, ask yourself, *"What other data do I need to either confirm or reject my nursing hypotheses?"* In each cluster group, document any additional data you would need to consider, but the information is not available. [Consider what you could obtain without a physician's order versus what would require a consultation.]

8. Now you are ready to write your nursing diagnoses. Examine the problem areas that you have identified. Select the areas that would apply to (have an impact on) Pearl's respiratory status. Document those diagnoses in the space provided.

     1.

     2.

     3.

     4.

     5.

9. What current Physician Orders does Pearl have in place that may have an impact on the nursing diagnoses that you identified in 8.? Include the number of the nursing diagnosis that the medical order applies to. What are the corresponding nursing activities that would apply, collaboratively and independently?

Nsg. Dx. #	Physician Orders	Nursing Activities/Orders

10. In the box below, document Pearl's arterial blood gases, as they occurred over time. Examine the trends, what do they indicate?

Values/Settings	ABG #1	ABG #2	ABG #3
O_2 Percentage:			
Resp. Rate:			
Mech. Vent. (Y / N):			
pH:			
$PaCO_2$:			
PaO_2:			
HCO_3:			
SaO_2:			
ABG Interpretation			

11. Based on your data cluster/problems, what do you now believe is/are Pearl's acute medical problems.

12. According to the existing data, what other multisystem involvement might be present in Pearl?

13. Focusing in on Pearl's respiratory status, does she primarily have a restrictive or an obstructive pulmonary problem at this time? Defend your choice.

14. Based on Pearl's age, activity level, history and other data, what complications is she most at risk of developing? What can you, as her nurse do, to help prevent these complications?

Case Study
The Case of Pearl M
Instructor Guide

*Note to teacher: This is a patient with a **restrictive** pulmonary problem*

Note: The Case of Pearl M. is a reality based case presentation. The data available may show evidence of multiple problem areas. The focus of today's case study, however, is the acute respiratory patient. Thus, most of the questions in this exercise will center around consideration of her respiratory status.

1. After you have read the Case Scenario of Pearl M., go through the data that is available on Pearl and underline or highlight all abnormal or suspicious data, beginning with the Recent History.

2. Once you have marked all abnormal/suspicious data, examine the data found in the **Initial Appraisal**. What abnormal or suspicious data did you find there? What general problem areas do these data fall into (e.g., cardiovascular, nutritional, psychosocial, etc.)?

3. Go to the clustering grid (Item #6). Document the general problem areas that you have already identified in the Initial Appraisal and the corresponding data that support it.

4. Based on your findings in 2. which part of your systematic bedside assessment should you perform first?
    Pulmonary, since it is the most severe sign at this time. Airway and breathing are often first
    priority assessments.

5. Now move on to Pearl's **Systematic Bedside Assessment. and Significant Labs and Other Tests**
    Examine the assessment data that you have selected as abnormal or suspicious. Enter these new findings onto the clustering grid.

> **NOTE**: You should be clustering data according to *critical cues*. All nursing diagnoses (and medical diagnoses) have critical cues that consist of a few pieces of data that strongly indicate the presence of a particular problem, disorder, or disease. For example, .the nursing diagnosis, *fluid volume excess* is supported by criteria such as: Intake > Output, edema, + JVD, and adventitious breath sounds (crackles). The medical diagnosis *acute renal failure* is supported by abnormally high BUN and Creatinine serum levels, and clinical manifestations of fluid excess. Your data can fit into more than one data cluster – many will.]

6. **Data Clustering:** Data clusters do not have to be placed in any order of priorities. Rather, it is suggested that you list them in order of how you discover them. Numbers are provided to help you identify clusters.

[Instructor: These data clusters are not comprehensive. Please add problem areas and data clusters as desired]

DATA CLUSTERING GRID		
	Abnormal/Suspicious Data	*Problem Area*
1	*Respirations appear rapid; rate of 28/min., labored and shallow. Adventitious breath sounds present. Abnormal arterial blood gases. Use of accessory muscles for breathing. Abnormal chest x-ray: patchy densities present in lungs bilaterally with large right pleural effusion and left lower lobe atelectasis.* Additional Data Needed: *sputum C & S results*	*Pulmonary*

	DATA CLUSTERING GRID	
	Abnormal/Suspicious Data	**Problem Area**
2	*Looks "worried"; First hospitalization; intermittent severe agitation of unknown origin; tracheostomy; unable to communicate with staff; unstable status* Additional Data Needed: *more, in-depth assessment data*	*Psychosocial*
3	*Tracheostomy tube; attempting to mouth words / sentences rapidly; appears frustrated with inability to talk. Unable to write notes legibly* Additional Data Needed: *evaluate site in left eye; evaluate hearing*	*Communication*
4	*Green secretions around tracheostomy tube; WBC 14.2; Differential: Segs: 9,500, Bands: 3,100, Lymphs: 1,000;* *Perineal erythema with small patches of white "cottage cheese-like" discharge present; intermittent severe diarrhea of unknown origin;* Additional Data Needed: *sputum and urine C & S; C & S of green tracheostomy drainage*	*Infection*
5	*Tachycardia of 100 - 120/min.; mild edema of extremities; abnormal chest x-ray: patchy densities observed in bilat. lungs; rapid weight gain. Intake > Output (1.5 liters) over past 48 hours* Additional Data Needed: ECG, jugular vein distention	*Perfusion*
6	*Urinalysis: cloudy appearance, protein 1+; culture and sensitivity pending; serum WBC: 14.2 perineal erythema with small patches of white "cottage cheese-like" discharge present; complaining of severe perineal burning; urine is foul smelling; BUN: 22, UN/Creatinine: 31* Additional Data Needed: results of urinalysis	*Elimination*
7	*Phosphorus = 2.3; Until recent rapid weight gain, had lost 7 pounds. Skin is hanging from body. Unable to swallow without coughing. Unable to eat; RBC = 4.14; Lymphs = 1,000; serum glucose = 176* Additional Data Needed: *serum albumin / prealbumin &/or transferrin; serum protein levels; urine urea nitrogen; prehospitalization weight pattern;*	*Nutrition/Metabolic*
8	*Several reddened areas over mid-back. mild edema in extremities; skin hangs loosely from body; tracheostomy tube in place; peripheral IV present; contusion over right ramus; perineal erythema* Additional Data Needed:	*Integumentary*

7. Once you have accounted for all of your abnormal / suspicious data through clustering, ask yourself, *"What other data do I need to either confirm or reject my nursing hypotheses?"* In each cluster group, document any additional data you would need to consider, but the information is not available. [Consider what you could obtain without a physician's order versus what would require a consultation.]

8. Now you are ready to write your nursing diagnoses. Examine the problem areas that you have identified. Select the areas that would apply to (have an impact on) Pearl's respiratory status. Document those diagnoses in the space provided.

> *1) Ineffective airway clearance*
> *2) Fluid volume excess (if severe, can cause pulmonary edema)*

3) *Infection (pneumonia can impair gas exchange, and plug up airway; fever causes hyperventilation)*
4) *Anxiety (can precipitate hyperventilation, increase work of breathing*
5) *Alteration in nutrition: less than body requirements (protein malnutrition weakens respiratory muscles)*

9. What current Physician Orders does Pearl have in place that may have an impact on the nursing diagnoses that you identified in 8.? Include the number of the nursing diagnosis that the medical order applies to. Based on these orders, what are the corresponding nursing activities that would apply, collaboratively and independently?

Nsg. Dx. #	Physician Orders	Nursing Activities/Orders
1	*Suction every 20-40 minutes. Portable chest x-ray; Up in chair TID; oxygen @ 30% per trach collar.*	*Consult with physician regarding suctioning order. Assess for need to suction q 20 - 30 min.; Suction as needed. Assure that order has been sent and procedure is done. Assist x-ray personal with positioning for x-ray. Assist patient as needed to get up in chair. Protect while sitting up.*
2	*Strict I & O*	*Assure that I & O records are accurately maintained. Monitor I & O trends. Alert medical team for imbalances.*
3	*Urine for UA and C & S* *Call House Officer for T > 101 (o)* *Tylenol 650 mg PO PRN q 4 hours* *Nystatin liquid 300 mg PO q 6 hours* *Nystatin Cream to peri area PRN q 4 hours*	*Assure that specimens are obtained correctly and in a timely manner. Monitor temp. q 4 hours; Administer Tylenol, and Nystatin as ordered and reassess for therapeutic and nontherapeutic effects. Report abnormal results of urine UA and C & S.*
4	*Cimetidine Liquid 300 mg PO q 6 hours.* *Mylanta 30 cc PO PRN*	*Administer drugs as ordered (through enteric tube). Monitor secretions for occult blood.*
5	*Full liquid diet. Pulmocare @ 75 cc/Hr.;* *Neutro-Phos Cap 1 T.I.D.;*	*Hold p.o. diet and consult with medical team regarding inability to swallow effectively. Administer Pulmocare as ordered. Assess placement every 4 hours. Turn off pump if H.O.B. is lowered. Administer drug as ordered. Monitor serum phosphorus, as obtained.*

10. In the box below, document Pearl's arterial blood gases, as they occurred over time. Examine the trends, what do they indicate?

	#1	#2	#3
%O:	*100%*	*50%*	*30%*
Respiratory. Rate:	*42*	*22-24*	*38*
Mech. Vent. (Y/N):	*No*	*Yes (1 hr following)*	*No (1 hr prior to transfer back to ICU)*

	#1	#2	#3
pH:	7.36	7.36	7.32
PaCO$_2$:	32	36	52
PaO$_2$	64	100	78
HCO$_3$:	26	25	30
SaO$_2$:	77%	96%	80%
ABG Interpretation:	Compensated respiratory. acidosis with hypoxemia. This ABG is unusual because her respiratory rate of 42/min. has been the _acute_ compensation mechanism prior to any increase in bicarbonate by the kidneys.	Resolution of acid-base imbalance. No hypoxemia. It is interesting to note that her PO$_2$ in only 100 on 50% oxygen. This reflects diffusion problems related to her acute pulmonary disorder.	Acute respiratory acidosis with hypoxemia (mild). Note that her breathing was rapid, shallow and labored.

11. Based on your data cluster/problems, what do you now believe is/are Pearl's acute medical problems?
    Possible pneumonia, atelectasis, pleural effusion, possible congestive heart failure, malnutrition, anemia, urinary tract infection

12. According to the existing data, what other multisystem involvement might be present in Pearl?
    Pulmonary, cardiac, renal, gastrointestinal

13. Focusing in on Pearl's respiratory status, does she primarily have a restrictive or an obstructive pulmonary problem at this time? Defend your choice.
    Restrictive. Her clinical presentation and supportive tests are consistent with a restrictive disorder.

14. Based on Pearl's age, activity level, history and other data, what complications is she most at risk of developing? What can you, as her nurse do, to help prevent these complications?
    [Instructor: This is meant to be a thinking piece for the students. I have included a few suggested answers.]
    She is at risk for multiple complications, particularly related to stasis: such as recurrent pneumonia, decubitus ulcers, thromboembolism, and urinary tract infection.

    The best way to prevent stasis related complications is to keep the patient as active as possible. Regular range of motion exercises, frequent turning, coughing and deep breathing, weight bearing through early ambulation, and sitting in chair. Prevent compression of vessels. This can be accomplished by careful positioning, preventing leg crossing. The bed needs to be maintained in a wrinkle free state and must be kept dry and clean. There are many more possible nursing interventions that can help prevent these problems related to fluid and nutrition.

Case Study
The Case of Thomas Bach

The Admission

Thomas Bach, a 68 year old farmer, is brought to the emergency room in acute respiratory distress. His wife gives the following brief history: Mr. Bach has had a 2 PPD smoking history habit for over 40 years and was diagnosed with COPD 15 years ago. She also relates the following medical history: Thomas was diagnosed with non-insulin-dependent diabetes (NIDDM) about 20 years ago. He has a 16 year history of ASHD and suffered a mild myocardial infarction 5 years ago. In addition, Mrs. Bach states that her husband has been taking the following medications at home: Diabinase, Isosorbide paste, Digoxin, Lasix, Slow-K, and - Theo-Dur. He has no known allergies to medications.

Mrs. Bach gives the nurse the following accounting of events leading up to his admission tonight: About two weeks ago, Thomas developed anorexia and dyspepsia which has increased steadily. Three nights ago he awoke with a sudden onset of severe shortness of breath which was relieved when he sat up in a chair. Over this time, she noticed that his legs had swollen up significantly. According to their home scales, Thomas had gained 6 pounds over the past two days despite his loss of appetite. Thomas indicates that he has had decreasing urine output for about 48 hours, which concerned him.

Initial Appraisal

Mr. Bach has just arrived from the emergency department. He has been placed in bed and you are preparing to perform an initial appraisal on him.

Mr. Bach is an elderly, Caucasian male who is sitting upright in bed, leaning forward with his hands on his knees. You note that his respirations are labored, with a distinctly prolonged expiratory phase. He has a loud, audible expiratory wheeze. His shoulders lift with every inspiration and you can see his neck muscles tightening with each breath. You note that he has nasal cannula in place but it has not yet been reconnected to an oxygen source.

Mr. Bach has thin, gray hair. His complexion is pale and lips are dark. His general health looks poor, with spindly arms and legs which lack both fat or significant muscle. You note that his lower legs are very edematous.

You walk over to the bed and introduce yourself, asking Mr. Bach to tell you his full name -- he complies. He is also able to tell you where he is, but does not know what day of the week it is. He has great difficulty talking with you due to his extreme shortness-of-breath and is able to say only two or three words at a time. His wife is at his bedside looking very anxious.

You note that he has an IV of D_5 NS infusing at a slow rate through a #20 intravenous catheter in his left hand.

Systematic Bedside Assessment

After getting Mr. Bach settled into the room and performing the initial appraisal, you decide to conduct a more in-depth head-to-toe assessment. Data collected is as follows:

V.S.:   BP = 160/90, P = 114 and slightly irregular, R = 32 & labored, T = 97.2 orally.

HEAD: Coloring pale, mucous membranes, earlobes, tongue and conjunctive are cyanotic. He is oriented to name and place, and cooperative. Positive jugular vein distention (JVD) is present while he is sitting up.

CHEST: **Pulmonary**: Breath sounds are distant and difficult to distinguish, particularly in bases. However, fine crackles are auscultated over bilateral bases, with coarse crackles and expiratory wheeze heard centrally. The A/P diameter of his chest is approximately 1:1 with little chest movement noted during breathing.
Cardiac: Heart sounds are very distant, rhythm is somewhat irregular. S_1 and S_2 are heard with difficulty, but you are unable to distinguish other heart sounds.

ABDOMEN: His abdomen is distended. He complains of discomfort when you palpate high in the upper right quadrant. Bowel sounds are present but hypoactive. No scars are noted on his abdomen.

PELVIS: A urinary catheter is in place. 50 cc of dark amber urine is noted in the urine collection bag. The urine specific gravity is = 1.036.

EXTREM.:   His legs are hairless below knees, with patchy brown areas noted. A healed ulceration noted on L. ankle. 4+ pitting edema is noted bilaterally on the lower legs. He has +radial pulses but you are unable to palpate pedal pulses due to the severe edema.

SKIN: His skin is warm, dry, and flaky. No areas of breakdown are noted. His general coloring & nail beds are dusky. His capillary refill is approximately 3 seconds.

Significant Labs and Other Tests

An **ABG** was drawn on room air. The results are as follows:

pH 7.34, $PaCO_2$ 65, PO_2 70, HCO_3 = 34, SaO_2 = 90%.

An **ECG** is performed, with the following interpretation:

Sinus tachycardia with occasional unifocal premature ventricular contractions (PVCs). The pattern is consistent with old inferior myocardial infarction.

A **Chest X-ray** is done, with the following results:

Fluid is noted, consistent with mild pulmonary edema. Cor pulmonale is evident.

The Case of Thomas Bach: Study Guide

1.   What risk factors does Thomas have? What disease processes are these risk factors associated with?

Risk Factor	Associated Disease Process
1)	
2)	
3)	
4)	

2.   Look at his at-home medications. What can you say about his preexisting medical conditions based only on his medication history?

3.   Based <u>only</u> on his admitting clinical presentation (data found in <u>The Admission</u> section), list at least three potential problems:

4.   Examine the data you have available in the <u>Initial Appraisal</u>. Reevaluate the tentative hypotheses you developed in Item 3. Which problems have been supported with this new data? Which problems are not supported? Which problems need more data before you can draw a conclusion?

    1)   Problems that are supported with new data:

    2)   Problems that are not supported with new data:

    3)   Problems that need more data:

5.   Based on the <u>Initial Appraisal</u>, at this time, what patient needs will you need to focus on FIRST? Defend your choice.

6.   It is time to finish analyzing available data. Examine the data found in the <u>Systematic Bedside Assessment</u> and <u>Significant Labs and Other Tests</u>. In the space provided, cluster all of the abnormal data that is available regarding Mr. Bach (beginning with his history and admission) into together that suggests a particular problem.

> **NOTE**: You should be clustering data according to *critical cues*. All nursing diagnoses (and medical diagnoses) have critical cues that consist of a few pieces of data that strongly indicate the presence of a particular problem, disorder, or disease. For example, the nursing diagnosis, *fluid volume excess* is supported by criteria such as: Intake > Output, edema, + JVD, and adventitious breath sounds (crackles). The medical diagnosis *acute renal failure* is supported by abnormally high BUN and Creatinine serum levels, and clinical manifestations of fluid excess. Your data can fit into more than one data cluster – many will.]
>
> Data clusters do not have to be placed in any order of priorities. Rather, it is suggested that you list them in order of how you discover them. Numbers are provided to help you identify clusters. Start with the data that, in your mind, readily stands out as belonging together to suggest a particular problem.

Abnormal Data Cluster	*Supported Problem Area*
Additional data needed:	
Additional data needed:	
Additional data needed:	

8. Based on patient history and assessment data, does Mr. Bach have an <u>acute</u> restrictive or obstructive pulmonary disorder? What symptoms would indicate this?

What do you believe is the underlying cause of this disorder?

9. Based on his history, does Mr. Bach have an <u>underlying</u> restrictive or obstructive pulmonary disorder?

10. Interpret Mr. Bach's initial arterial blood gas. Based on his medical history, what can you say about the significance of this ABG? Why?

11. Which of the following respiratory related nursing diagnoses best applies to Mr. Bach's current status?

    _____ Ineffective Airway Clearance:

    _____ Impaired Gas Exchange:

    _____ Ineffective Breathing Pattern:

12. Is Thomas experiencing any multisystem effects that may be in any way attributed to some degree to the patient's pulmonary disorder (acute renal failure, ARDS, cor pulmonale, etc.)?

13. List a minimum of FIVE Expected Patient Outcomes you would use to evaluate Mr. Bach's pulmonary status:

    1)
    2)
    3)
    4)
    5)

14. List a minimum of FIVE Collaborative Interventions appropriate to your patient's pulmonary status (drugs, respiratory therapy, mech. vent.):

    1)
    2)
    3)
    4)
    5)

15. List a minimum of FIVE Independent Nursing Interventions the nurse is performing that impacts on this patient's pulmonary status:

    1)
    2)
    3)
    4)
    5)

CONGRATULATIONS – YOU HAVE COMPLETED
THE CASE OF THOMAS BACH

The Case of Thomas Bach:
Instructor Guide

*[This is a patient with an **obstructive** pulmonary history]*

1. What risk factors does Thomas have? What disease processes are these risk factors associated with?

Risk Factor	Associated Disease Process
1) NIDDM	*Heart disease, peripheral vascular disease, renal dysfunction, peripheral neuropathies, loss of vision, and many others*
2) ASHD	*Angina, myocardial infarction, congestive heart failure, and others*
4) Smoking	*COPD, lung cancer, and others*
5) COPD	*Cor pulmonale, congestive heart failure, ventilatory insufficiency and failure, oxygenation insufficiency and failure, and others*

2. Look at his at-home medications. What can you say about his preexisting medical conditions based only on his medication history?

    His Diabinase suggests that he has NIDDM. His Isosorbide paste suggest that he has a history of angina. His Digoxin and Lasix suggest that he has congestive heart failure. The Slow-K is added as typical prophylactic therapy against hypokalemia and Digoxin toxicity related to his Digoxin and Lasix therapy. These drugs all reconfirm the history given by Mr. Bach's wife.

3. Based <u>only</u> on his admitting clinical presentation (data found in <u>The Admission</u> section), list at least three potential problems:

    1) fluid volume excess (congestive heart failure)
    2) myocardial infarction
    3) renal dysfunction / failure
    4) exacerbation of COPD

4. Examine the data you have available in the <u>Initial Appraisal</u>. Reevaluate the tentative hypotheses you developed in Item 3. Which problems have been supported with this new data? Which problems are not supported? Which problems need more data before you can draw a conclusion?

    Instructor – the answers placed here will depend on what the students writes in item 3. The following answers are based on the suggested answers.

    1) Problems that are supported with new data:
        Fluid volume excess (congestive heart failure) has the strongest cluster of critical cues.

    2) Problems that are not supported with new data:
        There is no data available to suggest a myocardial infarction.

    3) Problems that need more data:
        Exacerbation of his COPD is always a possibility. It will require more data collection to rule out an acute pulmonary condition, particularly pneumonia. Based on his history, one cannot rule out renal dysfunction without further evaluating laboratory data.

5. Based on the Initial Appraisal, at this time, what patient needs will you need to focus on FIRST? Defend your choice.

> *[Instructor: This is a thinking question. Students have the opportunity to think critically about their decision.] His cardiopulmonary status is the best answer. Respiratory status or cardiovascular status would be acceptable. Cardiopulmonary system is essential to life. Failure of either is associated with rapid deterioration and eventual death if not assessed in a timely manner and treated effectively.*

6. It is time to finish analyzing available data. Examine the data found in the Systematic Bedside Assessment and Significant Labs and Other Tests. In the space provided, cluster all of the abnormal data that is available regarding Mr. Bach (beginning with his history and admission) into together that suggests a particular problem.

> **NOTE**: You should be clustering data according to *critical cues*. All nursing diagnoses (and medical diagnoses) have critical cues that consist of a few pieces of data that strongly indicate the presence of a particular problem, disorder, or disease. For example, .the nursing diagnosis, *fluid volume excess* is supported by criteria such as: Intake > Output, edema, + JVD, and adventitious breath sounds (crackles). The medical diagnosis *acute renal failure* is supported by abnormally high BUN and Creatinine serum levels, and clinical manifestations of fluid excess. Your data can fit into more than one data cluster – many will.]
>
> Data clusters do not have to be placed in any order of priorities. Rather, it is suggested that you list them in order of how you discover them. Numbers are provided to help you identify clusters. Start with the data that, in your mind, readily stands out as belonging together to suggest a particular problem.

Abnormal Data Cluster	*Supported Problem Area*
+ JVD, wet lungs (crackles), peripheral edema, decreased urine output, hepatic tenderness, BP 160/90, P 114/min., rapid weight gain, cyanosis, severe shortness of breath, chest x-ray: mild pulmonary edema and cor pulmonale, previous MI Additional data needed: *ECG, CVP (if available)*	*Fluid balance problem (excess), cardiovascular origin*
Fine crackles: bilateral bases. Coarse crackles and expiratory wheeze present. ABG: compensated respiratory acidosis with mild hypoxemia. Resp. rate = 32/minute, labored and slightly irregular; long history of COPD. Chest x-ray shows mild pulmonary edema. Coloring dusky and pale. Prolonged expiratory phase. Oriented to name and place. Additional data needed: *Serial ABGs, WBC, RBC*	*Pulmonary problem: chronic and acute*
[There are several other potential problem areas that do not have adequate data to draw any conclusions: nutrition, renal are the two most obvious] Additional data needed:	

8. Based on patient history and assessment data, does Mr. Bach have an acute restrictive or obstructive pulmonary disorder? What symptoms would indicate this? *He has an acute restrictive disiease process.*

> *He has a clinical presentation consistent with fluid volume excess (including pulmonary edema). He has many symptoms: wet lungs (crackles), + JVD, , hepatic tenderness, decreased urine output and others. In addition, his chest x-ray confirms mild pulmonary edema*

What do you believe is the underlying cause of this disorder? *congestive heart failure*

9. Based on his history, does Mr. Bach have an <u>underlying</u> restrictive or obstructive pulmonary disorder?
   Obstructive. He has a positive history for COPD. His general appearance and clinical presentation are all consistent with an obstructive disease.

10. Interpret Mr. Bach's initial arterial blood gas.
    Compensated (chronic) respiratory acidosis with mild hypoxemia

    Based on his medical history, what can you say about the significance of this ABG? Why?
    While he will need to be observed closely until the his pulmonary edema is corrected, his ABGs look adequate with the exception of a slightly low pH. COPD patients are commonly in chronic respiratory acidosis and mild hypoxemia. The nurse will want to pay particular attention to his mentation. If he becomes confused, agitated, or overly drowsy, his ABG levels may be moving beyond his acceptable limits. His ABG will need to be monitored closely until his fluid status is stabilized and his pulmonary edema has subsided.

11. Which of the following respiratory related nursing diagnoses best applies to Mr. Bach's current status?
    Currently, he has some involvement with all three nursing diagnoses. Typically, it is difficult to accurately separate these apart in complex pulmonary patients. One could argue for either of the first two nursing diagnoses. Of more importance is the students reasons for deciding.

    _____ Ineffective Airway Clearance:
    Has adventitious lung sounds. Is at risk for this particularly in light of the presence of pulmonary edema secondary to left heart failure

    _____ Impaired Gas Exchange:
    Not a priority problem at this time He IS at high risk, however. Currently his ABGs are consistent with respiratory insufficiency not respiratory failure

    _____ Ineffective Breathing Pattern:
    Rate of 34, labored. The acute aspect of this problem should resolve with correction of his pulmonary edema. His respirations may chronically be somewhat labored, however.

12. Is Thomas experiencing any multisystem effects that may be in any way attributed to some degree to the patient's pulmonary disorder (acute renal failure, ARDS, cor pulmonale, etc.)?:
    His cardiovascular system is affected. His chest x-ray shows pulmonary edema and cor pulmonale. He is in heart failure. He is also at risk for development of acute renal failure should his third spacing cause a functional hypovolemic shock episode associated with decreased BP. His renal status will need to be observed closely. In addition, his nutritional and immune status should be thoroughly evaluated. His appearance suggests that he may be malnourished, which could complicate his recovery.

13. List a minimum of FIVE Expected Patient Outcomes you would use to evaluate Mr. Bach's pulmonary status:
    1) *Improved breath sounds*
    2) *ABG within acceptable limits for patient*
    3) *States decreased or usual level dyspnea (absence of dyspnea may be unrealistic in COPD)*
    4) *Usual mental status*
    5) *Absence of pulmonary edema by x-ray*

14. List a minimum of FIVE Collaborative Interventions appropriate to your patient's pulmonary status (drugs, respiratory therapy, mech. vent.):
    1) *Monitor ABGs, SpO_2 (pulse oximetry)*
    2) *Oxygen therapy - Low concentration 2-3L*
    3) *Drug therapy - Lasix, Aminophylline*

3) *Drug therapy - Lasix, Aminophylline*
4) *Digoxin Level possible (to R/O toxicity)*
5) *Possible nebulizer pulmonary treatments via IPPB*

15. List a minimum of FIVE Independent Nursing Interventions the nurse is performing that impacts on this patient's pulmonary status:

1) *Increase head of bed for comfort*
2) *Monitor respiratory status frequently*
3) *Turn and deep breathe (possible cough) every 1-2 hours*
4) *Encourage adequate hydration through close monitoring of I to O balance, urine output > 30/hr; strict I & O.*
5) *Balance rest/activity to decrease metabolic demands.*

CONGRATULATIONS – YOU HAVE COMPLETED
THE CASE OF THOMAS BACH

Case Study
The Case of Raymond Sinclair

Raymond Sinclair, 76 years of age, was transferred to a regional medical center with the chief complaint of severe shortness of breath and acute respiratory distress. Apparently Mr. Sinclair had only been home from the hospital for approximately one week after being treated for salicylate toxicity and pneumonia, requiring mechanical ventilation. When he was discharged home from his previous admission, he was considered to be in satisfactory condition. According to a relative, yesterday Mr. Sinclair developed rapid onset shortness of breath. He became diaphoretic, had an increased cough and developed a "wild look in his eyes". His relative also states that he "always looks like this right before he has one of his bad breathing spells". An ambulance was called and Mr. Sinclair was taken to a local rural hospital and then rapidly transferred to the Medical Center with oxygen therapy flowing at 2 liters/minute.

He arrived at the Medical Center Emergency Department (ED) at 2200. The Emergency Department staff documented that crackles and coarse rhonchi were auscultated throughout his lung fields. Pulse oximetry would not register. His skin was cold and clammy. He was alert and oriented. Following STAT ABGs, he was intubated and placed on a Bear V mechanical ventilator. Initial ventilator settings were: Mode: Assist/Control, Rate: 12, FiO_2: 100%, Tidal Volume: 750 mL. No PEEP or PSV was used.

STAT arterial blood gases drawn in the ED were:

2200 - pH = 7.12, PCO_2 = 75, PO_2 = 40, HCO_3 = 23.5, SaO_2 = 55.4%
2254 - pH = 7.17, PCO_2 = 68, PO_2 = 50, HCO_3 = 23.8, SaO_2 = 74%
2400 - pH = 7.28, PCO_2 = 50, PO_2 = 75, HCO_3 = 24.2, SaO_2 = 88% (2 hours post-mechanical ventilation)

STAT Medications administered in the ED included:

D_5W at a keep vein open rate via a #20 intravenous catheter in his left hand
Solumedrol 250 mg IV
Brethine 0.25 SQ
Lasix 40 mg (which was repeated X 1 after 10 minutes) for a total of 80 mg

Vital Signs ranges in the Emergency Department:

BP = <u>178 - 212</u> , P = 118 - 139, R = 34 - 40/minute, pulse oximetry SpO_2= non-registered to 84%.
113 - 148

PAST MEDICAL HISTORY

Mr Sinclair has a history of severe COPD, cor pulmonale, hypertension, and TIA (transient ischemia attacks). 5 years ago he developed pancreatitis which was treated medically. He also has an old left hip fracture. Medications he takes at home on a regular basis include: Theophylline, Lasix, Isordil, KCl, and Albuterol inhaler. He denies use of alcohol but has a long history of smoking.

Other Significant Data Obtained at Admission

STAT Chest X-ray: Large infiltrate in left lower lobe. Cor pulmonale noted.
STAT ECG: Evidence of inferior myocardial infarction of uncertain age, with changes consistent with recent extension.

Laboratory Data obtained on day of admission:

Glucose - 255	WBC = 25.3
BUN - 30	RBC = 4.88
Creatinine - 1.8	Hgb = 14.1

Albumin -2.0

Phosphorus - 1.8

Sodium - 142

Potassium - 4.4

Chloride - 103

CO_2 - 27

Osmolality - 298.08

Anion Gap - 16.37

A/G Ratio - 1.45

BUN/Creatinine - 16.96

Hct = 41.9

Platelets = 413

Lymphocytes = 3.8 %

Significant Progress Notes:

The following are exerpts from Mr. Sinclair's Physician Progress Notes:

1. **3 days following admission:** Echo is positive for myocardial infarction with recent extension. Mechanical Ventilator settings currently @:

    SIMV @ 10/minute, FiO_2 of 35%, Tidal Volume of 750 mL, PS of 10 cmH_2O

2. **5 days following admission:** Poor air movement present with continued wheezing heard bilaterally. Failed extubation yesterday: PaO_2 dropped to 68 and $PaCO_2$ increased to 70. Minute ventilation increased to 13 L/minute. Required reintubation and placed on mech. vent. at previous ventilator settings. Tracheostomy is planned to enhance clearance of secretions. Considering initiating IV nitroglycerine PRN for increased systolic blood pressure. Renal function remains borderline. To continue observing closely.

3. **Clinical dietetics consult:** 5' 11", 170 #. Albumin remains low at 2.0. Dubhoff placed, and tip is located post-pylorus. Recommend initiating Isocal HN at 90 mL/Hr. Will schedule a calorie count and urine urea nitrogen (UUN) to evaluate nitrogen balance.

Laboratory Data obtained following admission

Day #2:

ABG: pH 7.35, $PaCO_2$ = 52, PaO_2 = 88, HCO_3 = 35, SaO_2 = 92%

On ventilator settings of: SIMV at 12/minute, TV of 750 mL, FiO_2 of 30%

Day #4:

ABG: pH 7.37, $PaCO_2$ = 54, PaO_2 = 86, HCO_3 = 34, SaO_2 = 90% [On vent. settings of SIMV of 8/minute, TV of 750 mL, FiO_2 of 28% and 10 cmH_2O of PS]

Day #7: WBC = 9.7, RBC = 3.61, Hg = 10.3, Hct = 31.3, Platelets = 267

The Case of Raymond Sinclair: Study Guide

1. What acute event triggered Mr. Sinclair's respiratory crisis?

2. Does Mr. Sinclair have a restrictive, obstructive or combination pulmonary problem? Explain.

3. Specify what clinical manifestations he was exhibiting which resulted in being intubated. (Include interpretation of his initial ABG)

4. Based on the clinical manifestations you listed in #3, which of the following reasons for initiation of mechanical ventilation applies to Mr. Sinclair's situation?

   _____Acute ventilatory failure

   _____Impending ventilatory failure

   _____Acute oxygenation failure

   _____Apnea

5. Why do you think his initial ventilator settings might have been ordered as they were?

6. Why are his subsequent arterial blood gases not <u>corrected</u>?

7. Considering the available data, explain the reason that he may have failed his extubation attempt.

8. What will be your nursing priorities in managing Mr. Sinclair's nursing care?

9. What will be your priority nursing diagnoses and expected patient outcomes (goals)?

	Nursing Diagnosis	*Expected Patient Outcomes*
1.		
2.		
3.		
4.		
5.		

10.   Considering Mr. Sinclair's history and present state, does he have multisystem dysfunction? If "yes", which systems are having problems? Briefly explain what data you base your answer on.

11.   Consider Mr. Sinclair's altered communication problem. What can be done to address this problem?

12. Let us for a moment assume that Mr. Sinclair requires positive end-expiratory pressure (PEEP) for some reason. What impact will this have on other body systems?

CONGRATULATIONS
YOU HAVE COMPLETED THE CASE

The Case of Raymond Sinclair
Instructor Guide
A Patient Requiring Mechanical Ventilation

[Note to the Instructor: This case is fairly rich in diverse data since the patient has multiple system dysfunction. There are a variety of different clinical questions that can be asked in addition to the ones provided here. Of particular interest are the implications of his renal and nutritional status on his outcomes.]

1.   What acute event triggered Mr. Sinclair's respiratory crisis?

       His clinical presentation is consistent with a recurrence pneumonia (large infiltrate in LLL, WBC of 25.3). His severe hypoxia, respiratory acidosis and increased oxygen consumption may have precipitated an extension of his inferior myocardial infarction.

2.   Does Mr. Sinclair have a restrictive, obstructive or combination pulmonary problem? Explain.

       He has a history of long standing obstructive disease with an acute onset of a restrictive disease (pneumonia). The combination of the two is a common cause of a deterioration from a chronic state of respiratory insufficiency into an acute respiratory failure.

3.   Specify what clinical manifestations he was exhibiting which resulted in being intubated. (Include interpretation of his initial ABG)

       ABG Interpretation: Acute respiratory acidosis with severe hypoxemia. His acid-base imbalance as well as his state of hypoxia were both life threatening. Acute ventilatory failure (pH = <7.30 with a PCO_2 = >50) and oxygenation failure (PaO_2 = <60) are both criteria for mechanical ventilation. He is fortunate that his body is still able to muster of its compensatory mechanisms as evidenced by his elevated BP, P and R..

4.   Based on the clinical manifestations you listed in #3, which of the following reasons for initiation of mechanical ventilation applies to Mr. Sinclair's situation?

       _X_   Acute ventilatory failure
       _____ Impending ventilatory failure
       _X_ Acute oxygenation failure
       _____ Apnea

5.   Why do you think his initial ventilator settings might have been ordered as they were?

       His Assist/Control Mode was implemented to allow him to reduce his work of breathing (a resting mode). His FiO_2 was initially placed on 100% as an emergency method to increase tissue oxygenation. When his post-intubation ABG comes back from the lab, this will be reduced as quickly as is feasible. Though high FiO_2 is contraindicated in a COPD patient, the ventilator will take care of apnea that may develop. First priorities are always A - airway, B - breathing, including oxygenation. They can wean his levels down when he has stabilized.

6.   Why are his subsequent arterial blood gases not corrected?

       "Normal" ABGs are relative in the COPD patients. His acceptable blood gas levels are those that he tolerates the best -- based on his usual base line values. Priorities are to provide for adequate PaO_2 levels and to correct his pH. Once they resolve his acute physiologic crisis, they will eventually want to return his PCO_2 and PaO_2 to their usual base lines. (This may be a PCO_2 of 50 or 60, if that is his usual, and a PaO_2 of >60)

7.   Considering the available data, explain the reason that he may have failed his extubation attempt.

       Several problems may have caused him to fail his weaning attempt. 1) the physician's may have attempted to wean him prematurely (before his acute problem had resolved sufficiently). 2) His nutritional status was poor. Poor nutritional status causes weakening of muscles, including the respiratory muscles. 3) If he was on Assist/Control mode for several days, his diaphragm would already have begun to atrophy, secondary to lack of use via positive pressure ventilation.

8.   What will be your nursing priorities in managing Mr. Sinclair's nursing care?

Increase his oxygenation status and improve his ventilatory status. Enhance his ventilation-perfusion relationship. He will require aggressive nutritional support to build up his protein and electrolyte status.

9.   What will be your priority nursing diagnoses and expected patient outcomes (goals)?

Included below is a partial listing of some of the possible major nursing diagnoses and their expected outcomes. It is suggested that the teacher add and alter this list as desired.

Nursing Diagnosis	*Expected Patient Outcomes*
1. Alt. in respiratory function:	1. Improved lung sounds
a) impaired gas exchange	2. ABG within acceptable limits for pt.
b) ineffective airway clearance	3. Usual respiratory rate, rhythm & depth
c) ineffective breathing pattern	4. Usual mental status
2. Alt. nutrition: less than body requirements	1. Albumin within acceptable limits for patient
	2. Serum electrolytes within acceptable limits for patient
	3. Usual weight ± 2 pounds
3. Decreased cardiac output	1. BP, P within normal limits for patient
	2. Usual mental status
	3. Urine output >30 mL/hr
4. Decreased tissue perfusion: cardiac	1. Cardiac rhythm - sinus rhythm with usual number & type of PVC
	2. Denies chest pain
	3. No further changes on ECG
	4. Cardiac enzymes within normal limits
5. [Other desired focus]	

10.   Considering Mr. Sinclair's history and present state, does he have multisystem dysfunction? If "yes" which systems are having problems? Briefly explain what data you base your answer on.

Yes, he has other systems that are being strained. 1) Lungs - severe COPD; 2) Heart - cor pulmonale and acute myocardial infarction and possible CHF; 3) Kidneys - BUN and creatinine levels are high, indicating a probable problem with kidney function.

11.   Consider Mr. Sinclair's altered communication problem. What can be done to address this problem?

The nurse needs to use patience in exploring ways to communicate with Mr. Sinclair. If he can write, communication may not prove to be much of a problem. However, particularly during the acute phase of an crisis such as he is experiencing, he may not be able to write. Minimally, the nurse may need to rely on asking simple "Yes" and "No" questions. Use of special picture or alphabet boards may also be explored when he is able to tolerate their use. Reading his lips is a common way to try to communicate. As the nurse becomes more familiar with him, she/he can often anticipate what is needed.

12.   Let us for a moment assume that Mr. Sinclair requires positive end-expiratory pressure (PEEP) for some reason. What impact will this have on other body systems?

PEEP lowers cardiac output by decreasing venous return to the heart. It also decreases perfusion to the organs in the abdomen and kidneys. Should he require PEEP to assist his oxygenation status, his multisystem dysfunctions may become further aggravated.

Arterial Blood Gas Analysis Exercise

Directions:

Classify the following arterial blood gases as: normal, acute (uncompensated), partially compensated, or chronic (compensated); metabolic or respiratory; acidosis or alkalosis; and degree of hypoxemia (mild, moderate, severe).

	pH	PCO$_2$	PO$_2$	HCO$_3$	Analysis
1	7.36	55	58	33	
2	7.54	19	82	19	
3	7.44	36	64	23	
4	7.16	82	63	27	
5	7.24	42	60	16	
6	7.48	56	53	42	
7	7.10	93	55	30	
8	7.52	42	80	35	
9	7.37	75	52	43	
10	7.24	43	66	18	
11	7.54	28	88	22	
12	7.15	15	120	8	
13	7.37	42	95	25	
14	7.26	23	88	8	
15	7.43	28	82	18	
16	7.26	16	90	8	
17	7.53	42	82	40	
18	7.36	23	88	13	
19	7.18	40	90	25	
20	7.26	77	56	34	

Arterial Blood Gas Analysis Exercise
Instructor Guide

Directions:

Classify the following arterial blood gases as: normal, acute (uncompensated), partially compensated, or chronic (compensated); metabolic or respiratory; acidosis or alkalosis; and degree of hypoxemia (mild, moderate, severe).

	pH	PCO_2	PO_2	HCO_3	Analysis
1	7.36	55	58	33	Chronic respiratory acidosis with moderate hypoxemia
2	7.54	19	82	19	Partially compensated respiratory alkalosis. No hypoxemia.
3	7.44	36	64	23	Normal acid-base balance with mild hypoxemia. Note that acid base status approaching respiratory alkalosis.
4	7.16	82	63	27	Acute respiratory acidosis with mild hypoxemia.
5	7.24	42	60	16	Acute metabolic acidosis with mild hypoxemia.
6	7.48	56	53	42	Partially compensated metabolic alkalosis with moderate hypoxemia.
7	7.10	93	55	30	Partially compensated respiratory acidosis with moderate hypoxemia.
8	7.52	42	80	35	Acute metabolic alkalosis with no hypoxemia present.
9	7.37	75	52	43	Chronic (compensated) respiratory acidosis with moderate hypoxemia.
10	7.24	43	66	18	Partially compensated metabolic acidosis with mild hypoxemia.
11	7.54	28	88	22	Acute respiratory alkalosis with no hypoxemia present.
12	7.15	15	120	8	Partially compensated metabolic acidosis with hyperoxemia. Consult team regarding reducing oxygen level.
13	7.37	42	95	25	Normal ABG
14	7.26	23	88	8	Partially compensated metabolic acidosis with no hypoxemia present.
15	7.43	28	82	18	Chronic (compensated) respiratory alkalosis with no hypoxemia present.
16	7.26	16	90	8	Partially compensated metabolic acidosis with no hypoxemia present.
17	7.53	42	82	40	Acute (uncompensated) metabolic alkalosis with no hypoxemia present.
18	7.36	23	88	13	Chronic (compensated) metabolic acidosis with no hypoxemia present.
19	7.18	40	90	25	This ABG should be questioned, as it does not make sense. It should be repeated.
20	7.26	77	56	34	Partially compensated respiratory acidosis with moderate hypoxemia.

PROBLEM SOLVING EXERCISES
Suggestions For Use

Problem Solving Exercises take about 1 to 1 ½ hours to complete, depending on the length of time students are given to discuss things in their small groups.

1. Do not inform students about the outcome focus. The object of the exercise is to assist in learning clinical problem solving. The first half of the exercise involves developing nursing hypotheses which require knowledge of disease processes. The second half of the exercise involves developing a plan of care based on available data base.

2. If possible, break students into groups of approximately 7-10. If not possible, the exercise can be done as a large group effort. Ideally, there are a variety of supportive texts available in the room (lab manuals, drug manuals, med/surg texts).

3. The instructor becomes the patient and presents the scenario, answering questions each group asks.

4. Each group is asked to decide (and agree) on 4 major patient problems based on the preliminary data.

5. Each group is given a sheet of paper to write down questions they wish to ask the patient. Students are told the questions should relate to data collection (e.g. history, physical exam, labs, etc.)

6. Begin the first round of questions. Each group is allowed to ask one question. They are told to ask what they consider to be the highest priority assessment question. Instructor answers, solely based on the instructor's data sheet. Instructor can indicate in provided space, when each bit of data is requested. If students ask for data not included in the provided data base - state "no data is available". Do not volunteer data. (It is a good idea to make notations of questions that students ask that are not present in the instructor data sheet – they can be examined later for possible incorporation into the scenario for its next use.

7. Let students discuss for brief time (about 5 minutes), the data they obtained from the first round of questions. Begin second round of questions, based on the data obtained in the first round. Each group is allowed one question. Again, ask for what they believe is the most important data to obtain.

8. Let students discuss new data base for brief time (5 minutes). Begin third (final) round of questions. Each group is able to ask two questions.

9. Students are then instructed to cluster their data, based on all of the data they have asked for. They can also be requested to write down any further data they wish they could obtain to help confirm their hypothesis.

10. The remainder of the exercise (nursing process) can either be done during the first 30 minutes of the next class period or could be done as a take home exercise. Either way, students are to use available resources to develop a plan of care based on their data base.

Problem Solving Exercise
The Case of Marie M

Directions: Appoint a scribe to be in charge of writing necessary information on index cards (or sheet of paper) in Task #2. Appoint a speaker to represent your group during the interactions.

INITIAL FRAME

Marie M, a 52 year old business manager, has been a patient on your floor for two weeks following a motor vehicle accident. In that accident, Marie sustained a mild concussion, a lacerated spleen, a fractured right femur, and multiple abrasions over her face and extremities. She has been in traction since her admission.

Prior to admission, Marie had been in relatively good health, missing very few work days over the past 5 years. She is a smoker and has been allowed to continue smoking while hospitalized. She has been treated for hypertension for the past eight years.

Currently, Marie is complaining of chest pain and dyspnea.

****

TASK #1:

Based only on the available data, develop a list of at least 4 possible health problems that Marie may be experiencing. [Use your reference texts as necessary]

1.

2.

3.

4.

5.

TASK #2: [The Scribe should have one index card or piece of paper]

Using the provided index card, write down: 1) questions you would ask Marie, 2) assessments you would perform, and/or 3) tests / procedures that you would like to see obtained in developing nursing hypotheses and her nursing plan of care. (We're talking critical cues here). Please confine yourself to 3 - 5 items on your card.

TASK #3:

Examine all of the available data up to this point. Cluster the data beginning with the most critical cues, into relevant conceptual patterns/problems. Use your resource books to help you understand the significance of data that you may be unfamiliar with OR if the information is not available in a book, ask an expert who can interpret the data with you.

CLUSTER #1:

CLUSTER #2:

CLUSTER #3:

CLUSTER #4:

CLUSTER #5:

TASK #4:

Based on the data that you have available, what do you now believe is Marie's acute health problem?

[END FIRST PROBLEM SOLVING SESSION]

Based on your decision in Task #4, consider **Frame #3**, on the next page. This frame is to be completed as directed by your teacher. Be prepared to actively participate in completing this problem solving session.

FRAME #3
[To be completed as in-class or out-of-class exercise]

TASK #5:

Based on Marie's history and assessment data base, decide whether her pulmonary problem(s) is/are restrictive, obstructive, or both. Defend your choice(s). [Use your textbook as your primary reference]

TASK #6:

Develop a list of appropriate nursing diagnoses based on your data clusters.

NURSING DIAGNOSES

1.

2.

3.

4.

5.

6.

7.

TASK #7:

In the space provided below, identify which of the respiratory related nursing diagnoses apply to Marie's situation. How will the nursing. diagnosis. statement need to be completed? Based on your choice(s), what **Expected Patient Outcomes (EPOs)** will you include to evaluate Marie's status relevant to that/those diagnosis(es)?

_____ Ineffective airway clearance R/T

EPO: Marie will maintain effective airway clearance AEB:

****

(continues on next page)

_____ Impaired gas exchange R/T

EPO: Marie will maintain adequate gas exchange AEB:

****

_____ Ineffective breathing pattern R/T

EPO: Marie will maintain an effective breathing pattern AEB:

TASK # 8:

What type of collaborative and independent nursing interventions will you include in your plan to successfully maintain or attain your EPOs? Keep in mind that your interventions ALWAYS need to include how you will measure each of the EPOs as well as actions that help you succeed in meeting them.

COLLABORATIVE INTERVENTIONS:)

1.
2.
3.
4.
5.
6.

INDEPENDENT NURSING INTERVENTIONS:

1.
2.
3.
4.
5.
6.
7.

[THIS COMPLETES THE CASE OF MARIE M.]

The Case of Marie M.
Instructor Guide

Directions: Instructor, please review instructions. Students can appoint a scribe to be in charge of writing necessary information on index cards in Task #2. Appoint a speaker to represent your group during the interactions.

INITIAL FRAME

Marie M., a 52 year old business manager, has been a patient on your floor for two weeks following a motor vehicle accident. In that accident, Marie sustained a mild concussion, a lacerated spleen, a fractured right femur, and multiple abrasions over her face and extremities. She has been in traction since her admission.

Prior to admission, Marie had been in relatively good health, missing very few work days over the past 5 years. She is a smoker and has been allowed to continue smoking while hospitalized. She has been treated for hypertension for the past eight years.

Currently, Marie is complaining of chest pain and dyspnea.

****

TASK #1:

Based only on the available data, develop a list of at least 4 possible medical problems that Marie may be experiencing. [Use your Reference Text as necessary]

1. *Myocardial Infarction*
2. *Pneumonia*
3. *Pulmonary Embolus*
4. *CHF / Pulmonary Edema*
5. *Pulmonary Contusion*

TASK #2: [The Scribe should have one index card]

Using the provided index card, write down: 1) questions you would ask Marie, 2) assessments you would perform, and/or 3) tests that you would like to see obtained in developing a differential diagnosis and her nursing plan of care. (We're talking critical cues here). Please confine yourself to 3 - 5 items on your card.

[Instructor – each round takes about 10 minutes. 5 minutes for student small group consideration of questions to ask and 5 minutes to answer student questions. Each group can ask 1 question. You can do as many rounds as can be fit into 10 minute increments. Student "thinking" time can be shortened to less than 5 minutes if necessary. If a group does not have a question ready, move on to the next group]

TASK #3:

Examine all of the available data up to this point. Cluster the data beginning with the most critical cues, into relevant conceptual patterns/problems. Use your resource books to help you understand the significance of data that you may be unfamiliar with OR if the information is not available in a book, ask an expert who can interpret the data with you.

CLUSTER #1: *L. Upper lobe infiltrate. R = 26. Coarse crackles & rhonchi over L. lung fields. Pleural friction rub present on left. Respirations =. labored & shallow (splinting noted). Restless & agitated. Lips & ear lobes = dusky. Mucus. membranes = dark. Breathing = labored and rapid. Coughing up thick, rusty colored secretions. Breathing on room air. ABG = pH = 7.49, PCO2 = 33, PO2 = 53, SaO2 = 90%, HCO3 = 26. Sharp, knife-like non-radiating l. chest pain. Worsens with breathing. Temp = 101.*

CLUSTER #2: *I & O Balance over past 24 hours: I = 4,625 mL, O = 2,732 (a 1,893 excess). Coarse crackles present L. lung fields. Respirations labored. Heart rate = 120/minute. BP = 156/88. Edema noted in R. leg. No IV running. No S3 or S4 auscultated. Cough is present.*

CLUSTER #3: *Abdominal. wound: 25% scattered areas healing by secondary intention. Slightly reddened and edematous suture line. WBC = 15.3, Polys = 80, Bands = 4.5, Lymphs = 6, Monos = 7. Coughing up thick, rusty colored secretions. Skin is hot and diaphoretic. Temp = 101 (o). Culture of pulmonary secretions = pending. Gm. Stain = clusters of Gm. Positive cocci.*

CLUSTER #4: *Abdomen is distended and tight. Bowel sounds are hypoactive in all 4 quadrants. No stool in three days. On regular diet, eating approx. 50% of diet consistently.*

CLUSTER #5: *Weight loss of 10 pounds since admission. On regular diet - consistently eating about 50%. Serum phosphorus = low at 2.8. No data on other nutritional parameters.*

TASK #4:

Based on the data that you have available, what do you now believe is Marie's acute medical problem?

Probable pneumococcal pneumonia

[END FIRST PROBLEM SOLVING SESSION]

[Instructor – this is a good place to quit if time is short. Students can either complete the remaining tasks outside of class or it can be picked up again on another class day. It works best, however, to continue with the students coming up with clusters and working out the plan of care]

Based on your decision in Task #4, consider Frame #3. This frame will be completed during the next class period or as instructed. Be prepared to actively participate during the next class time, in completing this problem solving session.

FRAME #3

[To be completed as in-class (or as independent study) exercise]

TASK #5:

Based on Marie's history and assessment data base, decide whether her pulmonary problem(s) is/are restrictive, obstructive, or both. Defend your choice(s). [Use your textbook as your primary reference]

Marie has a clinical presentation typical of a restrictive pulmonary problem. The data base does not support an lower airway obstructive disorder. The following clinical presentation is typical of restrictive patient: Rapid, shallow respirations. Pneumonia is a major cause of acute restrictive problems. Her crackles are consistent with restrictive and the rhonchi represent the increased secretions in larger airways typical of pneumonia. Her ABG is typical of alveolar hyperventilation with hypoxia which occurs with pneumonia.

Instructor Problem List -- based on data:

PROBLEM LIST:

1. *Tachypnea, shallow respirations*
2. *Abnormal ABGs: Acute respiratory alkalosis with hypoxemia*
3. *Chest pain*
4. *Fluid volume excess*
5. *Tachycardia*
6. *Acute infection*
7. *Weight loss of 10 pounds since admission*
8. *Hypophosphatemia*
9. *Hypoactive bowel sounds, no stool in 3 days*
10. *Cough, producing thick, rusty colored secretions*

NURSING DIAGNOSES

Develop appropriate nursing diagnoses:

1. *Impaired gas exchange*
2. *Pain*
3. *Infection*
4. *Fluid volume excess*
5. *Alt. in nutrition: less than body requirements*
6. *Pot. ineffective airway clearance*
7. *Alt. in elimination: bowel r/t constipation*

TASK #7:

Which of the respiratory related nursing diagnosis apply to Marie's situation? [*Ineffective airway clearance, impaired gas exchange, ineffective breathing pattern*]. How will the Nursing. Diagnosis. statement need be completed? Based on your choice of appropriate respiratory nursing. diagnosis., what **Expected Patient Outcomes (EPOs)** will you include to evaluate Marie's status relevant to that/those diagnosis(es)?

Choose which diagnosis(es) is/are appropriate. Complete the nursing diagnosis statement and list EPOs in the space provided.

[Instructor: the following are some suggestions for possible respiratory related nursing diagnoses. These can be manipulated as desired]
****

__X__   *Pot. for* Ineffective airway clearance R/T *copious, thick secretions, ineffective cough associated with infectious process.*

EPO: Marie will maintain effective airway clearance AEB:
a)   *lung sounds clear or improved*
b)   *able to clear own secretions*

****

__X__   Impaired gas exchange R/T *alveolar hyperventilation AEB respiratory alkalosis, hyperpnea.*

EPO: Marie will maintain adequate gas exchange AEB:
a)   *Arterial blood gases within acceptable range*
b)   *Absence of dizziness, tingling sensations in extremities*

****

 X   Ineffective breathing pattern R/T *pain*

EPO: Marie will maintain an effective breathing pattern AEB:
a)   *Respirations: normal rate, rhythm, depth*

TASK # 8:

What type of collaborative and independent nursing interventions will you include in your plan to successfully maintain or attain your EPOs? Keep in mind that your interventions ALWAYS need to include how you will measure each of the EPOs as well as actions that help you succeed in meeting them.

COLLABORATIVE INTERVENTIONS: *(Partial list of possible orders)*

1.   *Antibiotic Therapy*
2.   *Oxygen Therapy*
3.   *Chest X-rays*
4.   *Labs: Arterial blood gases, CBC with diff.,* Sputum for gram stain & culture
5.   *IV fluid orders*
6.   *Diet orders*
7.   *Incentive spirometry*

INDEPENDENT NURSING INTERVENTIONS: *(Partial list of possible interventions)*

1.   *Cough and deep breathe every 1-2 hours*
2.   *Turn every 2 hours while on bed rest*
3.   *Monitor for therapeutic and nontherapeutic effects of drug therapy*
4.   *Encourage fluid intake*
5.   *Monitor intake and output*
6.   *Monitor temperature, respirations and pulse q 2-4 hours during acute phase*
7.   *Monitor for clinical manifestations of hypoxemia*

[THIS COMPLETES THE CASE OF MARIE M.]

FACULTY GUIDE: HISTORY/ASSESSMENT DATA
The Case of Marie M.

Directions: The following script is used as follows: As student "small groups" ask for information, the instructor reads the specific corresponding data. If a student question asks for specific information within one data cell, the instructor should read the entire cell. The "Requested Data" column is used to check off the data as students request it. You might want to check off using a pencil so that this form can be used repeatedly.

PARAMETER / TEST	Requested Data	DATA
Neurologic Related:		
Neuro Status:		Restless and agitated. Fully oriented at this time.
Oxygenation Related:		
Chest X-Ray:		Left upper lobe infiltrate noted. Enlarged heart noted.
ABGs:		STAT ABGs are drawn: pH = 7.49, $Paco_2$ = 33, PaO_2 = 53, SaO_2 = 90%, HCO_3 = 26
Pulse Oximetry:		SpO_2 = 88 to 90%
Lung Sounds:		Coarse crackles & rhonchi over L. lung fields. A pleural friction rub is present on left. Respirations. are labored & shallow (splinting).
Skin Coloring		Nail beds: slightly dusky. Lips and ear lobes: dusky. Mucous. Membranes = dark.
Oxygen Therapy		No oxygen is in place at this time.
Secretions:		Coughing up thick, rusty colored secretions
Cardiac Related:		
ECG:		Sinus Tachycardia. Rate: 120, P-R interval = 0.14 sec., QRS Int. = 0.04 sec., rare unifocal PVC noted. Non-specific T-wave changes.
Cardiac Enzymes:		CPK MB bands = <5% ; LDH_1 > LDH_2 , both are WNL.
Heart Sounds:		S1, S2, a soft murmur is auscultated
Vital Signs:		BP = 156/88, P = 124, R = 26, T = 101
Integument Related:		
Skin / Mucous Membranes:		Skin is hot and diaphoretic. Edema of R. leg is noted. No skin breakdown noted. Coccyx area is reddened.
Laboratory Related:		
Cultures / Gm. Stain:		Culture: Pending; Gram Stain: Clusters of Gm. + cocci.

PARAMETER / TEST	Requested Data	DATA
CBC with differential:		CBC findings = WBC = 15.3, Hgb = 13.2, HCT = 43, Polys = 80, Bands = 4.5, Lymphs = 6, Monos = 7.
Comfort Related:		
PAIN Specifics:		Sharp, knife-like non-radiating left chest pain. Worsens with breathing.
Signs Of Distress		Facial expression is tense. Breathing appears labored and rapid. Is restless in her bed
Fluid and Electrolyte Related:		
IV Fluids:		An intermittent infusion device is present in right arm for administration of IV meds
I & O:		Past 24 hours: Intake 4,625 mL, Output = 2,732 mL
Serum Electrolytes		Na = 140, Cl = 102, K = 3.8
Other:		
Height and Weight		Height = 5 ft. 3 in, Weight = 165#.
Current Meds:		Cimetidine. Tylenol #3 for pain.
Incision Site:		75% approximated. Primary intention wound. 25% scattered areas healing by secondary intention. Slightly reddened and edematous suture line. Small amount of serous drainage.
PTT:		PTT: Patient: 27.2 seconds/ Control: 26.4
Neck Veins:		Unable to assess, short neck and obesity
Abdomen:		c/o of abdomen being sore to palpation.
Past History:		Smoking history of 1 PPD for 30 years. Occasional use of alcohol. History of mild hypertension. No other medical history.
Allergies:		No known allergies
Other:		
Other:		

CLINICAL FOCUS: RESPIRATORY PROCESS

Student Name: _____

Date: _____

Patient Initials: _____: Room/Bed #: _____;

Admission Date: _____; Today's Date: _____.

Age: _____; Gender: _____;

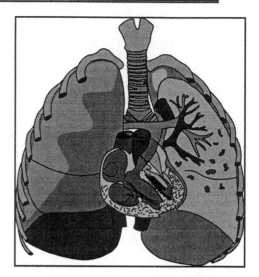

Admission Diagnosis(es): _____

_____.

Surgery &/or major Problems: _____

ASSESSMENT

1. Patient History
   A. Risk Factors:
      1) Pre-existing:

      2) Hospitalization related:

2. Cardiopulmonary Assessment

   A. Respiratory Assessment:

   B. Cardiac Assessment (if appropriate):

3. Supportive Data

    A. Laboratory (ABG, RBC, Hgb):

        DATA   **INTERPRETATION (significance)**

    B. Other (x-ray, scans, etc.):

        DATA   **INTERPRETATION (significance)**

4. What other data, not currently available, would you ideally like to obtain to strengthen your data clusters?

5. What drugs is your patient receiving that might directly or indirectly influence his/her respiratory status?

Drug	Classification	Effects	Significance/ Influence

ANALYSIS

6. Based on the data you have collected, choose which respiratory related nursing diagnoses best reflects this patient's actual or potential needs:

_____ *Ineffective airway clearance*
Supportive data cluster:

_____ *Impaired gas exchange*
Supportive data cluster:

_____ *Ineffective breathing pattern*
Supportive data cluster:

PLANNING

7. Based on your nursing diagnoses, what evaluative criteria can you use to evaluate the status of diagnoses?

8. List the physician orders currently written on your patient that may, in some way, impact on his/her respiratory status:

9. List at least 5 independent nursing interventions that could be realistically ordered for this patient to improve his/her respiratory status:

EVALUATION

10. Examine the Evaluative Criteria that you wrote in item # 7. Which criteria did this patient meet during your clinical day? Which criteria were not met? For those that were not met, what alternative nursing interventions could be implemented?

Criteria met:

Criteria NOT met:

Criteria   **Alternative Nursing Intervention**

DISCHARGE PLANNING NEEDS

11. What type of teaching or other activities need to be planned with this patient and/or family in anticipation for transfer or discharge?

PART III

CELLULAR OXYGENATION

PART III. CELLULAR OXYGENATION

Take Home Cases (THC)

     Cellular Oxygenation (Module 7)   99

     Shock States (Module 8)   101

Case Studies / Exercises

     The Case of Mr. Jones   103

     The Case of Nancy T.   107

Clinical Focus: Cellular Oxygenation   110

Take Home Case
Module 7: Cellular Oxygenation

Student name:_____   Date:_____

Directions:
       Using the appropriate reading assignment, complete the following questions or statements using complete sentences.

****

SITUATION: I. M. Hurt was recently involved in a motor vehicle crash. He obtained multiple internal injuries, and a collapsed lung. His Glasgow Coma Scale (GCS) score upon arrival to the University Medical Center was three.

Section one:
1.   Which component of oxygenation is Mr. Hurt's primary problem?

Section two:
2.   To assess Mr. Hurt's pulmonary gas exchange, what information is need?

Section three:
3.   Arterial oxygenation can be assessed by evaluating cardiac output, _____, arterial oxygen content, and autonomic nervous system innervation.

Section four:
4.   If Mr. Hurt's lactate level is elevated, how many molecules of ATP is he producing?

Section five:
5.   Mr Hurt's experiencing ventilation-perfusion mismatching. This leads to a condition called _____?

Section six:
6.   Explain why an increase in mixed venous oxygenation saturation (SVO_2) is not always a good thing.

Take Home Case
Cellular Oxygenation
Instructor Guide

1. Primary gas exchange

2. Degree of pnemothorax (how much surface area is comprised?). How healthy is the uninjured lung? What is his hemoglobin level? What is his oxygen saturation?

3. Autoregulation

4. Two

5. Hypoxemia

6. An increased SVO_2 level indicates that oxygen is not being used at the cellular level. This may mean that supply exceeds demand (a good thing!) or that a state of dysoxia exists where cells are unable to use the oxygen due to a metabolic problem (a bad thing).

Take Home Case
Module 8: Shock States

Student name_____ Date_____

Directions: Using the appropriate reading assignment, complete the following questions or statements using complete sentences.

****

Situation: Ms. Mays was shot in her abdomen during a robbery attempt.

Section one:
1.   For which type of shock state is she most at risk?

Section two
2.   A decrease in urinary output is noted.

2.   Describe the compensatory mechanism associated with decreased urinary output in this case.

Section three:
3.   What other clinical findings do you expect?

4. Complete the following table to describe hemodynamic findings associated with hypovolemic shock:

Hemodynamic parameter	Abnormal finding (elevated or decreased)
right arterial pressure (RAP)	
cardiac output (CO)	
pulmonary artery wedge pressure (PAWP)	
pulmonary artery pressure (PAP)	
systemic vascular resistance (SVR)	

Section four:

5.   What is the major treatment strategy for Ms. Mays?

6.   The goal of treatment is to obtain a hemoglobin level of_____.

Take Home Case
Module 8: Shock States
Instructor Guide

1.   transport

2.   ACTH > aldosterone > sodium and water retention > ADH > Reabsorption of water in kidney tubules.
      Renin is secreted in response to low blood volume > vasoconstriction

3.   cool, pale skin
      low blood pressure
      tachycardia

4.

Hemodynamic parameter	Abnormal finding (elevated or decreased)
right arterial pressure (RAP)	decreased
cardiac output (CO)	decreased
pulmonary artery wedge pressure (PAP)	decreased
pulmonary artery pressure (PAP)	decreased
systemic vascular resistance (SVR)	increased

5. packed red blood cells (RBC)
    surgery to correct the bleeding

6. 12g/100ml.

Case Study
The Case of Mr. Jones

Mr. Jones is a 78 year old admitted 3 days ago for a small bowel obstruction (SBO). The SBO did not resolve by medical interventions (NPO, NG tube) so he was taken to the operating room for a colectomy.

It is now 1 AM. You are working nights and have just entered Mr. Jones' room to perform you initial shift assessment on him.

He is sleeping when you enter the room. You awaken him to obtain his vital signs which are: BP 100/50, HR 110, R 20, T 100.8 F. You check his midline abdominal incision: it is intact and some old bloody drainage is noted. You verify the placement of his NG tube, drawing back apple-green drainage during aspiration. You note there is 500 mL in the NG collection chamber. His IV is patent with Lactated Ringers infusing at 75cc/Hr. His urinary catheter is intact. There is 50 mL in the urinary drainage bag.
****

1.   **Which data may be significant clues suggesting a possible fluid balance problem?**

2.   **What additional data would you like to obtain that would help you develop a hypothesis?**

3.   **Based on the initial data, what working nursing diagnosis would you suggest?**

4.   **What might be the medical diagnosis?**

5.   **What type of IV fluid orders would you anticipate?**

      CRYSTALLOIDS?   If yes, would he need isotonic solution, hypotonic, or hypertonic solution and why?

      BLOOD? If "yes", would he most likely receive whole blood or packed red blood cells? Why?

      If he received one unit of <u>whole blood</u>, you would credit his intake record with _____ mL. You would anticipate that his Hct would increase ___ - ___% and his Hgb would increase ___ - ___mg/dL within ____ - ____ hours?

If he receives one unit of <u>packed red cells</u>, you would credit his intake record with ___ - ___mL. You would anticipate that his Hct would increase ___ - ___% and his Hgb would increase ___ - ___mg/dL within ___ - ___ hour(s).

His blood will need to be hung with which type of IV fluid as a flush?

What gauge IV needle is the minimum desirable gauge? _____. Why?

6.   **If he receives blood, how will you need to alter your nursing care?**

7.   **As his fluid problem is being addressed, what expected patient outcomes will you be monitoring?**

The Case of Mr. Jones
Instructor Guide

Note: This is a Patient with a Fluid Balance Problem

Scenario

Mr Jones is a 78 year old admitted 3 days ago for a small bowel obstruction. The SBO did not resolve by medical interventions (NPO, NG tube) so he was taken to the operating room for a colectomy.

It is now 1 AM. You are working nights and have just entered Mr. Jones' room to perform you initial shift assessment on him.

He is sleeping when you enter the room. You awaken him to obtain his vital signs which are: BP 100/50, HR 110, R 20, T 100.8 F. You check his midline abdominal incision: it is intact and some old bloody drainage is noted. You verify the placement of his NG tube, drawing back apple-green drainage during aspiration. You note there is 500 mL in the NG collection chamber. His IV is patent with Lactated Ringers infusing at 75cc/Hr. His urinary catheter is intact and there is 50 mL of urine in the drainage bag.

****

1. **Which data may be significant clues suggesting a possible fluid balance problem?**
    a. *Age: >65 have decreased total body fluid weight; they have decreased thirst mechanism and have decreased renal function. They are at increased risk for dehydration secondary to smaller fat stores.*
    b. *Temp: For every degree temp. increase, 15% more fluids are needed to maintain balance.*
    c. *Hospital L.O.S.: 3 days of: NPO, NG tube draining, small bowel obstruction with 3rd spacing.*
    d. *Post-op abdomen: Risk for 3rd spacing.*
    e. *Dec. BP, Inc. HR, Inc. T -- Sx of dehydration*
    f. *500 mL NG drainage ; color green, NOT red*
    g. *IV at 75/Hr*
    h. *50 mL of urine*
    i. *Abdominal dsg. dry/intact so not bleeding*

2. **What additional data would you like to obtain that would help you develop a hypothesis?**
    a. *Specific Gravity*
    b. *Serum osmolarity (nl 385 - 395) -(if serum osmo was 310 then there is less fluid than solute) --can indicate if pt. needs fluid replacement (high osmolarity = concentrated)*
    c. *Previous shift's I & O balance. Remember that dec. U/O = a protective mechanism!*
    d. *Expected blood loss from surgery - can see if might account for deficit*
    e. *Labs: Hct, Hgb*
    f. *If had a central venous line could run a CVP on him. If had hemodynamic monitoring available could check cardiac output and PAWP.*
    g. *Weight: 1 kg = 1 Liter of fluid*
    h. *What are his usual vital signs? They may always look like this.*

3. **Based on the initial data, what working nursing diagnosis would you suggest?**
    Fluid volume deficit: (defining characteristics: Decreased BP, Increased HR, Increased Temp, Decreased U/O, increased Hct)

4. **What might be the medical diagnosis?**
    Dehydration - secondary to third spacing and expected blood loss (EBL) from surgery

5.   **What type of IV fluid orders would anticipate?**
      CRYSTALLOIDS?   If yes, would he need isotonic solution, hypotonic, or hypertonic solution and
            why?
      Types of fluid:
      Isotonic solutions *(e.g., 0.9% NS, LR) approximate normal serum osmolarity. Therefore, fluids will
            not shift and intravascular volume is expanded. Rx: dehydration, shock states.*
      Hypotonic solutions *(e.g., 0 .2 NS, 0.45 NS, D_5 & water). Have a low osmolarity -- therefore will shift
            water into intracellular (into cells) spaces. Rx: Used to hydrate pt.; prevent dehydration,
            increase urine output.*
      Hypertonic solutions *(e.g., D_5NS, D_{10}). Have a high osmolarity. Fluids will shift out of the cells and
            into extracellular spaces. Not as commonly used. Rx: water intoxication - to force fluid
            from cells.*

      ANSWER: *Yes. He would most likely receive isotonic solutions. His clinical presentation suggests a
            need for increased intravascular volume! The rate will need to be increased.*

      BLOOD? If "yes", would he most likely receive whole blood or packed red blood cells and why?

      Whole blood Vs. Packed Cells: *Since he does not have signs of hemorrhage, he will most likely
            receive one unit of PRBC.*
      Whole Blood: *Volume: 500 mL. 1 unit should increase a patient's Hct 2-3% and Hgb 1mg/dL.
            within 12 - 24 hours. Is used when volume is needed.*
      PRBC: *Volume: 200 - 250 mL. 1 unit should increase Hct 3-4% and Hgb 1.3mg/dL within 6 hrs.
            Used when blood loss is not a problem, anemia, pts. with fluid volume overload problems.
            He will need to have normal saline flush available.
            A # 18 gauge needle is the smallest desirable gauge size. A smaller size can cause breakage
            of the red blood cells as they squeeze through the lumen. This can reduce the desired effects
            of the blood as well as cause an increase in release of $K+$ from the cells.*

6.   **If he receives blood, how will you need to alter your nursing care?**
            -Increased frequency of VS
            -Monitor for S/S transfusion reactions
            -Give over 2 - 4 hours

7.   **As his fluid problem is being addressed, what expected patient outcomes will you be
monitoring?**
            -Increased U/O to >30 cc/Hr
            -Lungs clear
            -CVP normal
            -BP, P = WNL for patient
            -Skin turgor normal
            -I = O
            -No edema
            *-Weight normal for patient $\pm$ 2 Kg * (this range will depend on individual patient situation)*

Suggest the following as Independent study:

8.   **Consider whether or not Mr. Jones would be a candidate for colloid therapy. Be sure to know what
     colloids are and what their uses are.**

9.   **What is albumin and what are its uses?**

Case Study
The Case of Nancy T

Nancy T., a 45 year old woman was admitted to the hospital from a state mental health facility. She had a history of COPD, cor pulmonale, and long standing bipolar disorder. She was transported to the ED for increasing dyspnea, nausea, and increased confusion.

Past Medical History
1) Hx of COPD
2) Hx of bipolar disorder
3) Hx of cor pulmonale
4) no known allergies
5) presently taking lithium and Theodur

Recent History
Her dyspnea began 48 hours ago and has worsened. In the ED (yesterday) she was noted to have tachycardia, diaphoresis, and diffuses wheezes bilaterally. An IV was initiated and she received IV Solu-medrol and Lasix for her heart failure. STAT adrenergic nebulizer breathing treatments were not helpful. Her initial ABGs were:

pH 7.30, $PaCO_2$ 58, PaO_2 72, HCO_3 33

Nancy was admitted to a medical floor. One hour after her transfer, she was found unresponsive, with increased diaphoresis, and labored respirations. A STAT ABG was ordered. Results were:

pH 7.19 $PaCO_2$ 61, PaO_2 75, HCO_3 34

Results of labs ordered in the ED were made available:

Na 118, Cl 95, K 3.5
Theophylline level=22mg/dl

She is intubated and transferred to the ICU

She enters a metabolic coma believed to be caused from liver failure secondary to Lithium toxicity. Her lithium level is 2.8 mEq/L. She is maintained on steroids to treat her COPD exacerbation. Her glucose is 352. She is treated with sliding scale insulin.

Presently her vital signs are: P=154, R=14 A/C, B/P 100/70
T=102.6 rectal. A sputum culture reveals pseudomonas. The decision is made to insert a pulmonary arterial catheter. Her initial pressures are:

RAP = 12
PAP = 38/22
PCWP = 30
CI = 2.0

Derived parameters are: **SVR = 630**
She is placed on Norcuran and Dobutamine and diagnosed with cardiogenic and septic shock.

The Case of Nancy T: Study Guide

1) Assess Nancy for signs of hypoperfusion.

2) Assess Nancy for presence of the inflammatory response.

3) Assess Nancy for hypermetabolic response.

4) Identify appropriate nursing diagnoses for Nancy.

The Case of Nancy T Study Guide:
Instructor Guide

[Instructor note: Since a case involving a trauma patient is discussed in the book, a case study is provided to demonstrate the development of multiple organ failure in a medical patient]

1) Assess Nancy for signs of hypoperfusion.

>   *PO_2 level*
>   *O_2 sat level*
>   *tachycardia*
>   *hypotension*
>   *CI 2.0*
>   *PCWP 30*
>   *PAP 38/22*
>   *SVR 630*

2) Assess Nancy for presence of the inflammatory response.

>   *fever (despite steroid use)*
>   *positive sputum culture*
>   *hyperglycemia (greater than expected due to steroid use)*

3) Assess Nancy for hypermetabolic response.

>   *hyperglycemia*
>   *tachycardia*

4) Identify appropriate nursing diagnoses for Nancy.

>   *High risk for Impaired gas exchange R/T pulmonary edema*
>   *Fluid volume deficit R/T vasodilation as evidenced by low SVR*
>   *Decreased cardiac output R/T ventricular failure, increased pulmonary vascular resistance, and vasodilating toxins*
>   *High risk for Alteration in Nutrition: Less than body requirements R/T decreased oral intake, catecholamine excretion, and insulin resistance*

Clinical Focus: Cellular Oxygenation

Student name:_____ Date:_____

Patient Initials:_____ Admission date:_____ Age:_____ Gender:_____

Admission diagnosis:_____

Surgeries/Procedures:_____

****

Assessment

1. Document any conditions that impair gas exchange.

   ventilation impairment_____

   diffusion impairment_____

   perfusion impairment_____

2. Document lab. values that reflect arterial oxygenation.

3. Is your patient in aerobic or anaerobic metabolism? Justify your answer.

Physical Examination

4. What findings indicate the functioning of the sympathetic nervous system?

5. What compensatory response is the patient exhibiting?

Interventions

6. What nursing interventions are you performing that increase oxygen consumption?

7. What nursing interventions are you performing that decrease oxygen consumption?

Analysis

8. List your priority nursing diagnosis related to cellular oxygenation.

<u>Diagnosis</u>   <u>Expected</u> <u>Patient</u> <u>Outcome</u>

PART IV

PERFUSION

Part IV. Table of Contents

PART IV. PERFUSION

Take Home Cases (THC)
Perfusion (Module 11)   115
Hemodynamic Monitoring (Module 12)   118
Electrocardiographic Monitoring and Related Cardiac Medications (Module 13)   121

Case Studies / Exercises
The Case of Hugh Neff   124
The Case of Mike Brown   130
Hemodynamic Parameter Practice   133

C. **Clinical Focus: Perfusion**   135

Take Home Case:
Module 11: Perfusion

Student name:_____ Date:_____

Directions:

Using the appropriate reading assignment, complete the following questions or statements using complete sentences.

****

Situation: V.E. Gunterman experienced crushing chest pain accompanied with diaphoresis and nausea during an administrative conference at an elementary school where she serves as an assistant principal. Ms. Gunterman has been diagnosed with acute Myocardial Infarction in the ED.

Section one and two:

> **Ms. Gunterman is experiencing hemodynamic instability. A pulmonary artery catheter has been placed through the right subclavian vena cava. Hemodynamic readings are as follows:**

Cardiac output: 3.2 L/min   Cardiac Index: 2.2 L/min./m2

Heart rate: 120 bpm   Stroke volume: 50 ml/beat

1. Normal cardiac output is_____. Normal cardiac index is_____.

2. In your opinion, which of these (cardiac output or cardiac index) is the most precise for determining cardiac functioning?

Briefly defend your position:

3. Explain the physiologic events contributing to the elevated heart rate. Hint: A compensatory mechanism is occurring.

Section three: The Frank-Starling Law

> **Ms.Gunterman's ECG and cardiac isoenzymes indicate that she has had an anterior M I. The contractility of her heart has decreased.**

4. Describe the effect contractility exerts on stroke volume.

Section four: Pressure, flow, resistance

5. In cardiovascular terms: "flow" refers to_____. "Pressure" refers to_____.
   "Resistance" refers to_____ .

6. Explain how blood pressure can change when considering these components.

Section five: Conditions that Affect Cardiac Output

> **Your patient's condition has stabilized. Medications have been given to block the sympathetic nervous system response to pain and injury.**

7. Differentiate the cardiovascular response to sympathetic and parasympathetic stimulation

8. Medications have been administered to decrease afterload. Decreased afterload is accomplished by_____ arterioles.

Section six: Assessments of Cardiac Output

9. Describe how the nurse can noninvasively assess for diminished contractility in this patient.

> **Ms. Gunterman remains stable. Afterload reduction is important to maintain as it reduces her myocardial oxygen consumption.**

10. What physical findings may indicate increased afterload and alert the nursing staff to intervene?

Take Home Case
Perfusion
Instructor Guide

1. 4.0 - 6.0 L/min   2.5 - 4.5 l/min/m2

2. CI

   Corrects for body size

3. The HR is increasing to compensate for a low CI.

4. Poor contractility decreases SV.

5. Flow=CO

   Pressure= blood pressure
   Resistance= afterload

6. B/P elevates with increased afterload and increased flow and decreases when these decrease.

7. SNS= increased HR
           increased contractility
           vasoconstriction
   ANS= opposite effect

8. Dilating

9. Level of consciousness, presence/degree of chest pain, tachycardia

10. Cool, clammy skin, increased B/P, decreased capillary refill

Take Home Case:
Module 12: Hemodynamic Monitoring

Student name:_____. Date:_____

Directions:

        Using the appropriate reading assignment, complete the following questions or statements using complete sentences.

Reading assignment: *High Acuity Nursing, 2nd ed.* - Modules 12, Hemodynamic Monitoring.

****

Situation: B.F. Goodrich has been admitted to the ICU with pulmonary edema, left heart failure, and intermitttent ventricular dysrhythmias. A pulmonary artery catheter will help the nurses and physicians plan interventions to enhance cardiac functioning.

Section one: The PA Catheter

1. Mr. Goodrich is experiencing acute heart failure. Explain how a pulmonary artery catheter will help the nurses and physicians plan interventions to enhance cardiac functioning.

Section two: Cardiac Output (CO)

2. Define CO:

        What is the equation for determining CO?

        What measurement references CO to size?

Sections three, four, five, and six:

3. Mr. Goodrich has clinical evidence of elevated left ventricular preload.

        Elevation of which of the following hemodynamic readings would indicate left-sided failure with no right-sided pathology (circle all that apply):

RAP   PAD   PAWP   RV pressure

Section seven:

4. A Nipride drip has been started to decrease the resistance the heart has to pump against. An arterial line has been placed for continuous blood pressure monitoring.

        Briefly describe the function of the arterial line.

Section eight:

5. Calculate the SVR for Mr. Goodrich using the following data:

    BP: 150/100   RAP: 14   CO: 3.5   SVR:

    Is this a positive finding that will enhance his cardiac status?

    Explain your answer:

Take Home Case
Module 12: Hemodynamic Monitoring
Instructor Guide

1. Allows determination of pressures in the heart as well as how much blood is pumped out by the heart. Health care providers can determine if interventions are returning pressures to normal and enhancing cardiac output.

2. The amount of blood ejected from the heart into the systematic circulation each minute.

$$CO = HR \times SV$$
CI

3. RAP would elevate if LHF is severe.
   RV pressure is not continuously monitored. It would be elevated if the RAP is high and LHF severe.
   PAD would be elevated.
   PAWP would be elevated.

4. An arterial line provides continuous monitoring of B/P, increased accuracy of B/P, more precise titration of fluids and medications, ability to obtain blood samples (including ABGs) without hurting the patient.

5. $SVR = \dfrac{(MAP-RAP) \times 80}{CO}$ $\dfrac{(150 + 200)}{3} = 116.6\ (MAP)$

   $\dfrac{(116.6 - 14) \times 80}{3.5} = 2345$

   This is elevated since normal SVR is 800-1200. This is a negative finding due to increased afterload the heart must pump against to eject blood.

Take Home Case
Module 13: Electrocardiographic Monitoring and Related Cardiac Medications

Student name:_____ Date:_____

Directions: Using the appropriate reading assignment, complete the following questions or statements using complete sentences.
****

Section one:
1. Movement of sodium into the cell occurs during the _____ phase of an action potential.

Section two:
2. Describe the mechanical event that corresponds with components of an EKG.

EKG Component	Mechanical Event
P wave	
peak of QRS to end of T wave	

Sections three - eight:
3. The rates (beats/minute) of the following heart rhythms are:

Normal sinus rhythm:_____   Sinus bradycardia_____

Sinus tachycardia:_____   Supraventricular tachycardia_____

Junctional tachycardia:_____   Ventricular tachycardia:_____

Section nine:
4. A patient develops premature ventricular contractions (PVCs). Explain the circumstances requiring close surveillance of PVCs.

Section ten:
5. If a patient develops a third degree heart block, will he need to be treated? Justify your answer.

Section eleven:
6. When a patient experiences a myocardial infarction, in lead II, what component of the ECG changes?

Section twelve:
7. Because of their deteriorating condition, a patient requires defibrillation. Briefly differentiate defibrillation from cardioversion.

Section sixteen
8. Why is it important to note if your patient is on Beta blocking drugs?

Take Home Case
Module 13: Electrocardiogram Monitoring and Related Cardiac Medications
Instructor Guide

1. Depolarization

2.

EKG Component	**Mechanical Event**
P wave	move to hear P wave
peak of QRS to cnd of T wave	arterial depolarization, ventricular depolarization, and repolarization

3. Normal sinus rhythm: <u>60-100</u>   Sinus bradycardia: <u><60</u>
   Sinus tachycardia: <u>100-150</u>   Supraventricular tachycardia: <u>150-250</u>
   Junctional tachycardia: <u>>100</u>   Ventricular tachycardia: <u>>140</u>

4. > than 6 PVCs/min
   couplet
   multifocal PVCs
   > 3 PVCs in a row

5. Yes, The atria and ventricles are not synchronized so cardiac output is minimal or absent.

6. The Q wave becomes deep and wide.

7. Cardioversion is synchronized to discharge during the firing of an ectopic impulse. Lower voltages are uscd. The patient may be alert and need analgesia prior to the cardioversion

8. Beta blocking drugs decrease heart rate, contractility and arterial pressure. They inhibit the SNS. They also prevent the patient from compensating during a myocardial infarction. In cases of resuscitation, the patient is less likely to respond to interventions.

Case Study
The Case of Hugh Neff

Mr. Neff, age 66, was admitted with a diagnosis of acute anterior MI.

Past Medical History
1) ASHD
2) MI 10 years ago
3) chronic bronchitis
4) hypertension
5) diabetes

Recent History

C/O increasing dyspnea x 1 week. Developed chest pain not relieved with nitroglycerin. Became diaphoretic and pale. He went into ventricular fibrillation in route to the hospital in the ambulance. Converted with defibrillation.

Initial Assessment

He has an IV with D_5W and 20 mEq KCL infusing in his right arm. Cardiac monitor shows sinus rhythm with unifocal PVCs. He is hard of hearing but does not wear a hearing aid. Pleasant demeanor and states, "I'm glad to be alive". Color is pale but no diaphoresis present.

Systematic Bedside Assessment

vital signs: B/P $\underline{130\text{-}150}$, HR 84-100, R 20-26/min T 99^4-99^8 oral
70-80

Head: GCS score 15, no JVD. O_2 at 2 liters per nasal cannula, mucous membranes pale and moist

Chest: Non-productive cough. Bilateral wheezes auscultated on expiration. respirations even and un-labored at rest. Increased with accessory muscle use on exertion. S_1 S_2 present. Soft systolic ejection murmur present.

Abdomen: Soft, non-tender. Positive bowel sounds. No liver enlargement.

Pelvis: Normal male genitalia. Urinary catheter draining yellow urine. No BM. Intake=3050 Output=1625 in last 24 hours

Extremities: Bilateral pedal pulses 1+ with Doppler. No edema. Moves extremities spontaneously.

Denies numbness, pain. Negative Homan's sign.

Laboratory Data (Abnormals only)

Serial CPK #1= 132   #2=5750   #3=8080
CPK-MB bands on #3=15
Glucose 155

EKG

Complete left bundle branch block thought to be masking acute changes secondary to MI. Unifocal PVCs at 5/minute.

Chest X-ray: Cor pulmonale. No infiltrates noted.

The Case of Hugh Neff Study Guide

Admitting Diagnosis:_____

Age: _____

1. **Pertinent Past Medical History**

2. **Events leading to admission**

3. **Rapid Focused Circulatory Assessment**

4. **Because the heart is part of the cardiopulmonary circuit, continue with a focused respiratory assessment:**

5. **Based on patient history and assessment data, does the patient have an oxygen demand problem or an oxygen supply problem? What signs, symptoms, history, or risk factors would support this?**

6. **Based on patient history, and assessment data, does the patient have a fluid volume excess or fluid volume deficit? Which of these conditions would Mr. Neff be at risk for? Justify your answer with supporting data.**

7. **Develop three priority clusters of data and derive appropriate nursing diagnoses for each cluster.**

CLUSTER #1:   **NURSING DIAGNOSIS/ES**
CLUSTER #2:   **NURSING DIAGNOSIS/ES**
CLUSTER #3:   **NURSING DIAGNOSIS/ES**

8. **List a minimum of FIVE Expected Patient Outcomes you would use to evaluate Mr. Neff's perfusion status:**

    1)

    2)

    3)

    4)

    5)

9. **List a minimum of FIVE Collaborative Interventions appropriate to Mr. Neff's perfusion status:**

    1)

    2)

    3)

    4)

    5)

10. **List a minimum of FIVE Independent Interventions the nurse can perform that will promote perfusion:**

    1)

    2)

3)

4)

5)

Hugh Neff Study Guide
Instructor Guide

Admitting Diagnosis:
Age:

1. **Pertinent Past Medical History**
    ASHD
    COPD
    previous MI
    hypertension
    diabetes

2. **Events leading to admission**
    increasing dyspnea
    unrelieved angina
    ventricular fibrillation

3. **Rapid Focused Circulatory Assessment**
    LOC: Awake and oriented
    Vital Signs: BP = $\underline{130 - 150}$, HR = 84 - 100, RR = 20 - 26, SpO2 = 90
     70-80
    Heart Sounds: $S_1 S_2$ present. Soft systolic ejection murmur
    Skin: Coloring is pale. Mucous membranes = pale and moist. Skin is dry.
    Urine Output: U/O = 1625 in last 24 hours (with I = 3050, a 1425 excess)
    Edema/JVD: Negative for JVD, No edema in extremities
    Pain: Denies numbness or pain at this time
    Hemodynamic readings (if available): None available
    Cardiac pattern (if available): Complete L. BBB which may be masking acute changes secondary to MI. Unifocal PVC at 5/minute

4. **Because the heart is part of the cardiopulmonary circuit, continue with a focused respiratory assessment:**

    Airway: patent
    Oxygen Therapy: @ 2 Liters per nasal cannula
    Breath Sounds: Bilateral expiratory wheezes.
    Breathing Pattern: Respirations are even and unlabored. Somewhat labored and use of accessory muscles on exertion.

5. **Based on patient history and assessment data, does the patient have an oxygen demand problem or an oxygen supply problem? What signs, symptoms, history, or risk factors would support this?**
    The patient has an oxygen supply problem. Hx of ASHD, hypertension, previous MI, and chronic bronchitis all decrease available oxygen supply and delivery. Bilateral wheezes, use of accessory muscles with activity, cor pulmonale on chest x-ray, and elevated CPK support present illness contributes to decrease supply. $SpO_2 = 90$

6. **Based on patient history, and assessment data, does the patient have a fluid volume excess or fluid volume deficit? Which of these conditions would Mr. Neff be at risk for? Justify your answer with supporting data.**
    Presently, he does not have either, no JVD, rales, peripheral edema. He is at risk for fluid volume excess because of his hypertension, cor pulmonale, and intake exceeding his output.

7. Develop three priority clusters of data and derive appropriate nursing diagnoses for each cluster.

CLUSTER #1: *Hx ASHD, s/p MI, angina, hypertension, diabetes, smoking history increasing dyspnea, episode of cardiac arrest with cardioversion, EKG showed bundle branch block probably masking acute EKG changes, CPK-MB=15, CPK#3=8080, PVC activity*
NURSING DIAGNOSIS/ES: *High risk for decreased cardiac output R/T pump failure*
CLUSTER #2: *s/p MI, Hx COPD, cor pulmonale, increasing dyspnea, intake greater than output, expiratory wheezes, non-productive cough, dyspnea on exertion*
NURSING DIAGNOSIS/ES: *High risk for fluid volume excess R/T pump failure*
CLUSTER #3: *Hx COPD, bilateral expiratory wheezes, mild labored breathing pattern with accessory muscle use on exertion*
NURSING DIAGNOSIS/ES: *Activity Intolerance R/T decreased surface area for oxygen exchange*

8. **List a minimum of FIVE Expected Patient Outcomes you would use to evaluate Mr. Neff's perfusion status:**
   1) *No edema*
   2) *No dysrhythmia*
   3) *No angina*
   4) *No change in responsiveness level*
   5) *B/P within normal range for patient*

9. **List a minimum of FIVE Collaborative Interventions appropriate to Mr. Neff's perfusion status:**
   1) *O_2 at 2 liters per nasal cannula*
   2) *Nitroglycerin prn angina*
   3) *Lidocaine protocol if PVCs worsen and patient exhibits signs of decreased CO*
   4) *Cardiac monitoring*
   5) *pulse oximeter*

10. **List a minimum of FIVE Independent Interventions the nurse can perform that will promote perfusion:**
   1) *HOB elevated*
   2) *planned rest periods*
   3) *maintain I&O, monitor trends*
   4) *monitor potassium and glucose*
   5) *treat pain and anxiety quickly using pharmaceutical as well as non-pharmaceutical means*

Case Study
The Case of Mike Brown

Present Illness:

Mr. Brown was brought to the hospital by his wife. He is 85 years old. When he awakened this morning, his right side was paralyzed and he had no sensation in his arm or leg. Mr. Brown was quickly evaluated in the ED and admitted into ICU.

Past Medical History:

Mr. Brown did not have any significant illness until 12 months ago when he started developing bilateral senile cataracts. He began to consume large quantities of alcohol as his eyesight worsened. Two months ago the cataracts were removed and lenses implanted. They said they were told he had high blood pressure at that time. Other than his feet swelling occasionally, he was in good health.

Current Medications:

Digoxin .25 mg qd po
Lasix 20 mg qd po
Procardia 10 mg po TID

Initial Assessment:

General Appearance: Responds to questions inappropriately. GCS score 14. B/P 180/100, HR 110 irregular, RR 22, T 100.0 degrees oral

Head: Face is flushed. Slight JVD noted at HOB 30 degrees.

Chest: Bilateral crackles auscultated. S_1 S_2 present. PMI shifted laterally. Systolic ejection murmur present. Atrial fibrillation on monitor.

Abdomen: Non-distended. Bowel sounds present all quadrants.

Pelvis: Voiding clear yellow urine per urinal.

Extremities: Peripheral pulses 2+ all extremities. Spontaneous movements left side. Right side flaccid.
****

Case Study Worksheet: Mr. Brown

1. What perfusion related laboratory test orders do you anticipate based on Mr. Brown's history?

2. Mr. Brown is in atrial fibrillation. Why could Mr. Brown be experiencing this rhythm? What are treatment alternatives for this rhythm?

3. What are priority nursing diagnoses for Mr. Brown?

****

Upon re-assessment you note the following:

Mr. Brown does not respond to verbal stimuli. He grunts when pressure is applied to his nailbeds. His left extremities no longer move spontaneously. Vital Signs: Respirations 10, deep with long expiratory phase. B/P 180/70, HR 68 irregular. Laboratory data is now available: K^+ 3.0 other electrolytes are normal, digoxin level 0.25 ng/dl.

****

4. What is the significance of this data related to perfusion?

The Case of Mike Brown
Instructor Guide

1. What perfusion related laboratory test orders do you anticipate based on Mr. Brown's history?

> *potassium level/electrolytes*
> *digoxin level*
> *BUN (to determine renal function, ability to metabolize digoxin, reaction to diuretic)*
> *clotting profile (provide baseline for heparin therapy)*

2. Mr. Brown is in atrial fibrillation. Why could Mr. Brown be experiencing this rhythm? What are treatment alternatives for this rhythm?

> *He could have beginning heart failure secondary to hypertension. The patient's dose of digoxin may be too low or the patient may be non-compliant. May also indicate digoxin toxicity. Verapamil may be administered if cardiac output is compromised. Patient could receive an extra digoxin dose if level is too low.*

3. What are priority nursing diagnoses for Mr. Brown?

> *High Risk for aspiration R/T increased ICP*
> *High risk for impaired swallowing R/T muscle weakness*

****
Upon re-assessment you note the following:
    Mr. Brown does not respond to verbal stimuli. He grunts when pressure is applied to his nailbeds. His left extremities no longer move spontaneously. Vital Signs: Respirations 10, deep with long expiratory phase B/P 180/70, HR 68 irregular. Laboratory data is now available: K^+ 3.0 other electrolytes are normal, digoxin level 0.25 ng/dl.
****

4. What is the significance of this data related to perfusion?

> *Potassium level is low. To prevent bradydysrhythymia anticipate administering KCL or a potassium sparing diuretic.*
> *Digoxin level is low, anticipate administration of digoxin to increase contractility.*
> *Pulse pressure has widened, decreased LOC, ICP may be increasing. Decreased cerebral perfusion*

Hemodynamic Parameter Practice Sheet

DIRECTIONS: Classify the following hemodynamic parameter trends as reflecting: Fluid Volume Deficit, Fluid Volume Excess, Normal fluid status, preload, contractility, and afterload status, and probable associated medical condition.

RAP	PAP	PAWP	CO	SVR	Analysis
a) 4	35/14	14	4.0	1853	
b) 16	40/25	25	2.0	1546	
c) 14	35/20	20	3.0	1511	
d) 22	54/32	30	3.0	2968	
e) 14	40/20	20	4.0	2000	
f) 10	35/15	18	10	300	
g) 5	40/25	15	7.0	780	
h) 8	40/25	23	3.2	1890	
i) 12	40/26	21	2.3	2086	
j) 3	12/6	6	3.13	1700	

Hemodynamic Exercise
Instructor Guide

a)   fluid volume excess, increased right ventricular preload, increased left ventricular preload, increased afterload (CHF)

b)   fluid volume excess, increased preload, decreased contractility, increased afterload (cardiogenic shock)

c)   fluid volume excess, increased preload, decreased contractility, increased afterload (hypervolemia r/o CHF)

d)   fluid volume excess, increased preload, decreased contractility, increased afterload (pulmonary hypertension with CHF)

e)   fluid volume excess, increased preload, normal contractility, increased afterload (pulmonary hypertension, hypervolemia)

f)   normal fluid volume, normal preload, increased contractility, decreased afterload (septic shock)

g)   normal fluid volume, normal preload, normal contractility, slightly increased right ventricular systolic pressure, normal afterload (early pulmonary hypertension)

h)   fluid volume excess, normal right ventricular preload, increased left ventricular preload, decreased contractility, increased afterload (left ventricular failure)

i)   fluid volume excess, increased preload, decreased contractility, increased afterload (CHF)

j)   fluid volume deficit, decreased preload, decreased contractility, increased afterload (hypovolemia)

l)   fluid volume excess, increased preload, decreased contractility, increased afterload (CHF)

Clinical Focus: Perfusion

Student name_____ Date:_____

Patient initials:_____ Admission date:_____ Age:_____ Gender:_____

Admission diagnosis:_____

Surgeries/Procedures:_____

****

Assessment

1. Documented cardiovascular disease:

2. Cardiac risk factors:

3. Alterations in cardiac output may manifest as changes in mentation, urine output, or GI function. Record patient data pertaining to these systems.

   <u>Neurological status</u>

       EMV score: Abnormal findings:

   <u>Renal status</u>

       UOP (include amount and time period):

       Is UOP normal for your patient ?   If not, explain variation:

   <u>Gastrointestional status</u>

       Bowel sounds: Abnormal findings:

4. Physical Examination

   An adequate cardiac output (CO) is essential to life. Determinants of CO are heart rate, preload, afterload and contractility. Evaluate the components of cardiac output by analyzing the following physical assessment data:

Component of CO	Physical Assessment	Normal	Patient Finding/ Value	Analysis
Heart rate	heart rate	60-100 bpm		
Preload	jugular neck veins	nondistended		
	ascites	absent		
	peripheral edema	absent		
	skin turgor	elastic		
	mucous membrane	moist		
	orthostatic hypotension	absent		
	dyspnea	absent		
	cough	absent		
	heart sounds	S1, S2		
Afterload	skin	warm, dry		
	blood pressure	120/80, 140/90		
	skin color	pink, black, brown, racial variations		
	wounds	adequate healing		
	nail beds	average thickness, nonbrittle		
Contractility	pulses	present moderate strength		
	cardiac pattern, if monitored	NSR		

5. Document the physician's interpretation of your patient's current ECG here:

If the ECG is normal, what nursing or medical interventions are you implementing to treat the problem?

6. Does the patient's chest x-ray show any cardiac abnormalities ? If so, describe:

7. List cardiovascular tests completed on your patient (i.e., cardiac catheterization, echocardiogram, Thallium scan, vascular doppler studies).

      Briefly explain abnormal findings:

      Intervention/Evaluation

8. Work up one of the following perfusion related nursing diagnosis on your patient. Write 3 EPOs and identify at least 3 independent and 3 collaborative interventions for the diagnosis.

      Activity intolerance, decreased cardiac output, fatigue, fluid volume excess, knowledge deficit, noncompliance, altered skin integrity, altered tissue perfusion, self care deficit

Nursing Diagnosis

1.

EPOs

1.

2.

3.

Interventions

Independent

1.

2.

3.

Collaborative

1.

2.

3.

9. Many hospitalized patients receive medications that exert their main effects on the cardiovascular system. Complete the following table on all of the cardiovascular drugs your patient is receiving.

Medication	Classification	Effect on heart rate	Effect on blood pressure	Effect on cardiac rhythm	Reason your patient is receiving this medication

10. Describe the most important intervention during clinicals this week to improve your patient's cardiovascular status.

Note: Your future employer may ask you to explain why you are a good candidate for employment. Are you skilled at assessing, intervening, and evaluating? Do you deliver above average nursing care? Here is your chance to practice describing your unique/valuable talents!

PART V

NEUROLOGIC

Part V. Table of Contents

PART V. NEUROLOGIC

Take Home Cases (THC)
    Responsiveness (Module 15)   141

Case Studies/Exercises
    The Case of Billy Bob   144
    The Case of Susan   149

Problem Solving Exercise (PSE): The Case of Mary Burns   153

Take Home Case
Module 15: Responsiveness

Student name:_____   Date:_____

Directions:

In narrative form, complete the following questions or statements based on the Module reading assignment. To better comprehend this material, it is best to answer the items in your own words rather than copying answers from the text. By doing so, you can evaluate what you actually understand.

Reading assignment: *High Acuity Nursing, 2nd ed.* -- Module 15: Responsiveness.

****

Situation: Mary M., a 63 year old female is brought to her local Emergency Department with symptoms of visual disturbances, severe headache, dizziness, and left sided paralysis. She is admitted with a diagnosis of possible stroke. Her daughter reports that Mary has a history of hypertension and was previously hospitalized for Transient Ischemic Attacks (TIA's). She is alert but lethargic. Her right pupil is larger than her left pupil. She is oriented to person, place, and the month of the year. She demonstrates left sided weakness, but is able to follow simple commands and move all extremities.

Section one:
1. Differentiate the two components of responsiveness, and form the above scenario what neurological findings represent the components of responsiveness?

Sections two and three:
2. Assume Mary's nervous system is intact, what physiologic compensatory mechanisms attempt to maintain adequate intracranial volume (ICV) in the face of increased intracranial pressure (ICP) according to the Monro-Kellie hypothesis?

3. If Mary's ICP is 18 mm Hg, and her BP = 80/50, calculate her CPP. Is this acceptable? Explain your answer.

Sections four and ten:

> Mary's condition is deteriorating. Her level of consciousness is decreasing and she begins to have respiratory distress. She demonstrates non-generalized seizure activity involving the left side of her face that last for one minute. She is intubated and placed on mechanical ventilation with the following settings:
> TV 800 mL, FIO$_2$ 40%, Assist control mode with rate of 12. Her postintubation ABC showed the following results: pH 7.32, PaCO$_2$ 55, PaO$_2$ 120, SaO$_2$ 98%, HCO$_3$) 3 25.

4. Are these blood gases acceptable? What vent changes are indicated?

Sections five, six, and seven:

5.   Mary's pupils are both dilated and non reactive to light. What are the possible causes of this finding?

Section ten:

6.   A subarachnoid screw and transducer is placed to monitor Mary's intracranial pressure (ICP). What are the limitations of this device?

Take Home Case
Module 15: Responsiveness
Instructor Guide

1. Content: follows simple commands
   Oriented to person, place, time

   Arousal: alert but lethargic

2. Brain volume, cerebral blood volume, and CSF will adjust to change in one of the three.
   In response to increased ICP: 1) CSF will shunt out of the subarachnoid space; 2) Auto regulation will either constrict or dilate cerebral blood vessels in response to a change in B/P or CO_2 or oxygen blood levels; 3) The brain will attempt to compress itself depending on the degree of available compliance.

3. The ABGs indicate respiratory acidosis. Acidosis promoted dilation of cerebral vessels and increased ICP. The vent settings should be changed to increase the rate enough to blow off CO_2 and return the pH to normal and decrease the CO_2 between 25-30.

4. Herniation due to uncompensated increase in ICP although unlikely due to her history, a drug overdose may cause dilated pupils.

5. CSF cannot be drained.
   Wave form becomes easily dampened.

6. $CPP = MAP - ICP$ $MAP = \dfrac{SBP + 2\,DBP}{3}$

   $60 - 18 = 42$ $\dfrac{80 + 100}{3} = MAP$

   Normal CPP is 80-100 mm Hg. This is extremely low. A CPP of <50 does not provide enough cerebral blood flow.

Case Study
The Case of Billy Bob
A Patient with a Responsiveness Problem of Structural Etiology

Billy Bob was involved in an altercation at the "Bashful Bandit" nightclub. He was assaulted on the head with an unknown blunt object. He fell onto the pavement after being struck. At the scene he was combative and aggressive. He answered questions appropriately. He was transported by ambulance. Billy's Glasgow Coma Scale score in the ED was 15. He is admitted to the ICU. Billy's breath smells of alcohol.

Past Medical History
1) Hypertension

Recent History
Saw physician 2 weeks ago for headaches. Diagnosed with hypertension and placed on Procardia. Billy did not get the prescription filled.

Initial Assessment
Primary Survey:

Airway:	No noisy respirations. Air movement present
Breathing:	Cheyne Stokes pattern.
Circulation:	Pulse present. No obvious bleeding. Skin cool and clammy.
Disability:	Lethargic, confused. Pupils unequal, react sluggishly. GCS score 12.
Vital Signs:	B/P = 100/70, HR = 102, R = 14, T = 99.0 oral

Systematic Bedside Assessment
Head: Laceration 5cm in length, 2cm in width, posterior head. No active bleeding at present. Negative JVD. Spider angiomas on face.

Chest: Vesicular breaths sounds bilaterally. Negative abrasions, contusions.

Abdomen: Hypoactive bowel sounds. Abdomen distended with ascites. Non-tender on palpation.

Pelvis: Voiding clear yellow urine per urinary catheter. Output **has decreased from 100cc to** 50cc in the last hour.

Extremities: Skin is cool and clammy. No obvious deformity. Multiple abrasions on forearms.

****

Laboratory data is now available.

ABGs on room air are:	pH = 7.34, $PaCO_2$ = 48, PaO_2 = 76, HCO_3 = 29, O_2 Sat = 94%,
Blood alcohol level:	300 mg/dl
Serum Osmolality:	310 mOsm/kg H_2O
Lactic acid level:	15 mg/dl
Electrolytes:	within normal limits
Hemoglobin:	12 g/dl
Hematocrit:	48%
Glucose:	180mg/dl

Other Tests:
Chest film is negative.
Head CT scan results are pending.

The Case of Billy Bob: Study Guide

1) **Past Medical History**

2) **Events Leading to Admission/Mechanism of Injury**

3) **60 Second Appraisal/Primary Survey**

4) **Based on the Primary Survey, at this time, what will you need to focus on as:**
    First Priority:

    Second Priority:

5) **Rapid Focused Cerebral Assessment**

6) **Derive an appropriate nursing diagnosis based on the clustered data in #5:**

7) **List a minimum of FIVE Expected Patient Outcomes you would use to evaluate this patient's responsiveness.**

8) **List a minimum of FIVE Collaborative Interventions appropriate to your patient's responsiveness level:**

9) **List a minimum of FIVE Independent Nursing Interventions appropriate to your patient's responsiveness level:**

The Case of Billy Bob Study Guide
Instructor Guide

1) **Past Medical History**
History of untreated hypertension. Admission B/P is low for a hypertensive patient. May reflect hypovolemia secondary to blood loss from head laceration or vasodilation secondary to alcohol intake.

2) **Events Leading to Admission/Mechanism of Injury**
Blunt trauma with unknown object at unknown force. Fell onto concrete after being struck. Possible shearing and compression forces. Age of patient may be important data to collect since elderly patients have a higher incidence of subdural hematomas due to cerebral atrophy and increased vessel fragility.

3) **60 Second Appraisal/Primary Survey**
ABCs intact. No immediate life/limb threatening event. Change in LOC noted. Decreased responsiveness. Particularly important in relation to history of lucid interval at scene. Unequal pupils and history of blunt trauma may indicate an arterial bleed (epidural hematoma)

4) **Based on the Primary Survey, at this time, what will you need to focus on as:**

First Priority: *Decreasing level of responsiveness. Protect airway. Have suction available. Place a nasopharyngeal airway since patient is alert enough to have intact gag reflex.*

Second Priority: *B/P 100/70 in a patients with hypertensive history. Urine output decreasing. Want to maintain MAP in order to maintain CPP.*

5) **Rapid Focused Cerebral Assessment**
    *ABGs indicate respiratory acidosis/cerebral vasodilation
    *blood alcohol level indicates vasodilation
    *Serum osmolality indicates blood loss
    *Hemoglobin is decreased indicating blood loss
    *Hematocrit is increasing indicating blood loss
    *Decreased GCS score indicating increased ICP

6) **Derive an appropriate nursing diagnosis based on the clustered data in #5:**

   High risk for injury R/T altered cerebral function as evidenced by altered pupillary response, acidosis, GCS score 12.

7) **List a minimum of FIVE Expected Patient Outcomes you would use to evaluate this patient's responsiveness.**

    1) No aspiration
    2) No further decrease in responsiveness
    3) Pupils will be equal and react briskly
    4) improvement in ABGs
    5) urine output 1mg/kg/hr

8) **List a minimum of FIVE Collaborative Interventions appropriate to your patient's responsiveness level:**

    1)osmotic diuretics (must be titrated carefully with blood administration due to blood loss)
    2)high flow oxygen
    3)anticonvulsant therapy

    4)packed red blood cell administration
    5)fluid restriction

9)   <u>**List a minimum of FIVE Independent Nursing Interventions appropriate to your patient's responsiveness level:**</u>
    1)HOB elevated 30 degrees
    2)keep head in neutral position
    3)avoid hip flexion
    4)avoid Valsalva maneuver
    5)decrease noise and environmental stimuli

Case Study
The Case of Susan

Susan, a 20 year old female was brought to the Emergency Department with slurred speech and ataxia. Her friends brought her to the hospital because she was acting funny.

Past Medical History

Not available.

Recent History

Not available.

Initial Assessment

The patient is restless. She is oriented to person only. She moves her extremities upon command but movements are weak. She is pale. While addressing the patient, the nurse notices a Valium bottle in her pocket. there is one tablet in the bottle. When questioned, the patient states she took "some" but will not give you a number.

Systematic Bedside Assessment

V.S.: B/P 100/60, HR 70, R 16 non-labored.

Head: Pale and diaphoretic. Negative JVD. Neuroassessment as above.

Chest: Fine crackles bilaterally in the lower lung fields. S_1 and S_2 present without extra heart sounds.

Abdomen: Patient complains of nausea. Abdomen soft with bowel sounds present.

Pelvis: No voiding since arrival.

Extremities: Hypoactive reflexes. Negative edema.

Skin: Skin is warm and dry. Capillary refill within 3 seconds.

The Case of Susan: Study Questions

1. How did the nurse assess arousal (Reticular Activating System)?

2. How could the nurse assess content (cerebral function)?

3. What physiologic responses can produce restlessness?

4. What additional neurologic data should the nurse collect?

5. Based on your understanding of Valium (students are allowed to use reference books), What vital sign changes should the nurse anticipate? How do these changes differ from those vital sign changes associated with increased ICP?

6. The nurse in this case study was fortunate to discover the cause of the patient's decreased responsiveness. What are other possible etiologies of decreased responsiveness? List symptoms that would be present for each etiology.

POSSIBLE ETIOLOGY	SYMPTOMS

The Case of Susan (Responsiveness) Case Study
Instructor Guide

Decreased Responsiveness of Metabolic Origin

1.   **How did the nurse assess arousal (Reticular Activating System)?**
      The nurse assessed the patient's response to verbal stimuli and degree of purposeful movement.

2.   **How could the nurse assess content (cerebral function)?**
      The nurse should assess orientation x 4 (to person, place, time, and reason for being at the hospital). Memory should be assessed as well as the patients verbal ability and behavior.

3.   **What physiologic responses can produce restlessness?**
      hypoxia
      anxiety
      pain
      hypoglycemia
      increased ICP
      drug induced response

4.   **What additional neurologic data should the nurse collect?**
      pupillary response
      gag reflex with suction available
      cranial nerve function

5.   **Based on your understanding of Valium (students are allowed to use reference books), What vital sign changes should the nurse anticipate? How do these changes differ from those vital sign changes associated with increased ICP?**
      Valium produces hypotension, bradycardia, and bradypnea. Increased ICP produces widening of the pulse pressure. Systolic B/P will increase while diastolic B/P decreases. Bradycardia will eventually occur. Ataxic breathing develops.

6.   **The nurse in this case study was fortunate to discover the cause of the patient's decreased responsiveness. What are other possible etiologies of decreased responsiveness? List symptoms that would be present for each etiology.**

Drugs	*needle tracks, nasal dust, dust under fingernails, dilated pupils*
Ethanol	*visual hallucination, tremors, palmar erythema, spider angiomas*
Trauma	*abrasions, ecchymotic areas*
Epilepsy	*incontinence, post-ictal behavior, slow response*
Cold	*inappropriate clothing for weather, chills, bradycardia*
Tumor	*cachexia, PMH, weight loss*
Infection	*fever, headache, nuchal rigidity*
Vascular	*slurred speech, hemiparesis*
Endocrine	*acetone smell, thick glasses, flushed, diaphoretic*

**Problem Solving Exercise
The Case of Mary Burns**

Part 1

INITIAL FRAME

Mary Burns, a 69 year old retired factory worker, has been a patient on your floor for three days. She was admitted one month ago for a right cerebrovascular hemorrhage (CVA). Mary spent 30 days in a neuro intensive care unit. She required mechanical ventilation initially due to a deep coma (associated with an admission Glasgow Coma Scale score of 3). Mary became responsive five days after CVA. Her discharge from the NICU was delayed due to difficulty weaning her from the ventilator. Mary has dysphagia, motor apraxia, and intermittent disorientation. Her left sided weakness is improving. Since the CVA, Mary has had an occasional generalized (grand mal) seizure.

Prior to admission, Mary was treated for hypertension with diuretic therapy. She is obese, approximately 50 pounds overweight. Today, the nursing staff is concerned about Mary's increasing edema and fever. She has diminished breath sounds in her lower lung fields (left diminished greater than right). She has dyspnea on exertion. Her legs have 3 + pitting and ascites is developing.

Task #1

Based only on the available data, develop a list of at least four possible etiologies for Mary's edema.

1.

2.

3.

4.

5.

Task #2

Using the provided index card, write down: 1) questions you would ask Mary, 2) assessments you would perform and/or 3) tests that you would like to see obtained in developing a differential diagnosis and her nursing plan of care. (Hint: you want to focus on critical cues). Confine your number of items on your cards to 3 to 5.

> [At this point, students/groups will be given the opportunity to ask questions from their index cards to develop a specific data base]

Note: This exercise is also listed in Part VI C 2 due to the complex nature of this case.

Task #3

Examine all of the available data up to this point. Cluster the data beginning with the most critical cues, into relevant conceptual patterns/problems. If available, use your reference books to help you understand the significance of the data that you may be unfamiliar with or, if the information is not available in a book, ask an expert who can interpret the data with you.

CLUSTER #1:

CLUSTER #2:

CLUSTER #3:

CLUSTER #4:

CLUSTER #5:

==

Task #4

Based on the data you now have available, what do you now believe is Mary's acute health problem?

This is the end of Part One of this exercise.

The Case of Mary Burns
Part II

Task #5

New Available Data:
Mary has the following tests run:

Prealbumin = 8 mg/dl (nl= > 16mg/dl); transferrin = 200mg/dl (nl = 230 = 320mg/dl).
Lymphocyte count = 20% with a WBC of 18,000. TLC = 3,600 (WNL).

Based on the existing data, a tentative diagnosis of malnutrition/hypermetabolism was made. What other information could you collect on your assessment or through laboratory testing that will confirm or refute this diagnosis? Identify 5 items.

1.

2.

3.

4.

5.

Task #6

Why was Mary at risk for a nutritional deficiency? Work with your group and list 3 reasons. Explain the relationship between the item and nutritional status.

Reason	Nutritional Relationship
1.	
2.	
3.	
4.	
5.	

Task #7

Develop a list of nursing diagnosis appropriate for Mary. Prioritize among these diagnoses. Describe the etiology and evaluate criteria for each diagnosis.

Priority #	Diagnosis	Etiology	Evaluative Criteria

[This ends the Case of Mary Burns]

PROBLEM SOLVING EXERCISES
Suggestions For Use

Problem Solving Exercises take about 1 to 1 ½ hours to complete, depending on the length of time students are given to discuss things in their small groups.

1. Do not inform students about the outcome focus. The object of the exercise is to assist in learning clinical problem solving. The first half of the exercise involves developing nursing hypotheses which require knowledge of disease processes. The second half of the exercise involves developing a plan of care based on available data base.

2. If possible, break students into groups of approximately 7-10. If not possible, the exercise can be done as a large group effort. Ideally, there are a variety of supportive texts available in the room (lab manuals, drug manuals, med/surg texts).

3. The instructor becomes the patient and presents the scenario, answering questions each group asks.

4. Each group is asked to decide (and agree) on 4 major patient problems based on the preliminary data.

5. Each group is given a sheet of paper to write down questions they wish to ask the patient. Students are told the questions should relate to data collection (e.g., history, physical exam, labs, etc.).

6. Begin the first round of questions. Each group is allowed to ask one question. They are told to ask what they consider to be the highest priority assessment question. Instructor answers, solely based on the instructor's data sheet. Instructor can indicate in provided space, when each bit of data is requested. If students ask for data not included in the provided data base - state "no data is available". Do not volunteer data. (It is a good idea to make notations of questions that students ask that are not present in the instructor data sheet – they can be examined later for possible incorporation into the scenario for its next use.

7. Let students discuss for brief time (about 5 minutes), the data they obtained from the first round of questions. Begin second round of questions, based on the data obtained in the first round. Each group is allowed one question. Again, ask for what they believe is the most important data to obtain.

8. Let students discuss new data base for brief time (5 minutes). Begin third (final) round of questions. Each group is able to ask two questions.

9. Students are then instructed to cluster their data, based on all of the data they have asked for. They can also be requested to write down any further data they wish they could obtain to help confirm their hypothesis.

10. The remainder of the exercise (nursing process) can either be done during the first 30 minutes of the next class period or could be done as a take home exercise. Either way, students are to use available resources to develop a plan of care based on their data base.

**Problem Solving Exercise
The Case of Mary Burns
Instructor Guide**

Part 1

INITIAL FRAME

Mary Burns, a 69 year old retired factory worker, has been a patient on your floor for three days. She was admitted one month ago for a right cerebrovascular hemorrhage (CVA). Mary spent 30 days in a neuro intensive care unit. She required mechanical ventilation initially due to a deep coma (associated with an admission Glasgow Coma Scale score of 3). Mary became responsive five days after CVA. Her discharge from the NICU was delayed due to difficulty weaning her from the ventilator. Mary has dysphagia, motor apraxia, and intermittent disorientation. Her left sided weakness is improving. Since the CVA, Mary has had an occasional generalized (grand mal) seizure.

Prior to admission, Mary was treated for hypertension with diuretic therapy. She is obese, approximately 50 pounds overweight. Today, the nursing staff is concerned about Mary's increasing edema and fever. She has diminished breath sounds in her lower lung fields (left diminished greater than right). She has dyspnea on exertion. Her legs have 3 + pitting and ascites is developing.

Task #1

Based only on the available data, develop a list of at least four possible etiologies for Mary's edema.

1. immobility, bedrest (fluid shift)

2. CHF association with hypertension

3. fluid overload (IV)

4. acute renal failure

5. third spacing secondary to low albumin

Task #2

Using the provided index card, write down: 1) questions you would ask Mary, 2) assessments you would perform and/or 3) tests that you would like to see obtained in developing a differential diagnosis and her nursing plan of care. (Hint: you want to focus on critical cues). Confine your number of items on your cards to 3 to 5.

[At this point, students/groups will be given the opportunity to ask questions from their index cards to develop a specific data base]

Task #3

Examine all of the available data up to this point. Cluster the data beginning with the most critical cues, into relevant conceptual patterns/problems. If available use your reference books to help you understand the significance of the data that you may be unfamiliar with or if the information is not available in a book, ask an expert who can interpret the data with you.

CLUSTER #1:

Dyspnea on exertion. Decreased breath sounds LLF with left > right. Small infiltrate in left LLF on x-ray. Right CVA. Hospitalized x 33 days.

CLUSTER #2:

Elevated WBCs. Fever. Decreased B/P. HR 110. On steroids. Hyperglycemic. Negative cultures.

CLUSTER #3:

Weight loss. On Sustacal 50cc/hr. per feeding tube. Decreased albumin. Decreased RBCs, hemoglobin, and hematocrit. On HCTZ. Hospitalized x 33 days. Right CVA.

CLUSTER #4:

Edema, hx of hypertension, CAD. In Atrial fibrillation. Elevated serum osmolality. Intake > output. On HCTZ and nifedipine

CLUSTER #5:

Hx of right CVA. GCS 14. On dilantin and decadron. Occasional seizure. In atrial fibrillation

Task #4

Based on the data you now have available, what do you now believe is Mary's acute health problem?
Third spacing secondary to low albumin

This is the end of Part One of this exercise.

The remaining tasks can be completed at this time, completed as an independent assignment, or continued at another class time.

The Case of Mary Burns: Part II

Additional data:

Mary has the following tests run:

Prealbumin = 8 mg/dl (nl= > 16mg/dl); transferrin = 200mg/dl (nl = 230 = 320mg/dl).
Lymphocyte count = 20% with a WBC of 18,000. TLC = 3,600 (WNL).

Prealbumin and tranferrin both indicate malnutrition. Total lymphocyte count (TLC) does not indicate compromised immunocompetence at this point.

Task #5

Based on the existing data, a tentative diagnosis of malnutrition/hypermetabolism was made. What other information could you collect on your assessment or through laboratory testing that will confirm or refute this diagnosis? Identify 5 items.

Visceral protein assessments: prealbumin, total lymphocyte count, albumin

Somatic protein assessments: arm circumference, creatinine height index

Fat stores: triceps skinfold thickness, weight loss

Task #6

Why was Mary at risk for a nutritional deficiency? Work with your group and list 3 reasons. Explain the relationship between the item and nutritional status.

Reason	*Nutritional Relationship*
Dysphagia	• Potential for aspiration
Motor apraxia	• Unable to remember how to feed self
Age	• Decreased pepsin, HCL, and lactose secretion. Decreased gastric mucous and motility
Drug therapy: 　Dilantin 　Decadron 　HCTZ	• Anticonvulsants decrease folate uptake • Increases cortisol secretion and pancreatic demands. • Promotes water and sodium retention 　　May produce K^+ deficiency
Obesity	• May be malnourished prior to CVA; decreased protein, increased fat stores

Task #7

Develop a list of nursing diagnosis appropriate for Mary. Prioritize among these diagnoses. Describe the etiology and evaluate criteria for each diagnosis.

Priority #	Diagnosis	Evaluative Criteria	Priority Neg. Actions
#1	Alt. in nutrition: less than body requirements r/t motor apraxia, dysphagia, hypermetabolism	1. weight within normal range for age, build and height 2. Serum labs within normal limits 3. triceps skinfold within normal limits	1. monitor for clinical manifestations of malnutrition 2. monitor % of meals eaten 3. asses causes of inadequate intake 4. implement measures to maintain adequate intake 5. monitor lab values and report abnormals

Priority #	Diagnosis	Evaluative Criteria	Priority Neg. Actions
#2	High risk for impaired skin integrity r/t decreased mobility	1. no skin breakdown 2. no redness or irritation	1. turn q 2 hours 2. massage bony prominences q 2 3. keep skin dry and clean 4. avoid shearing activities
#3	Infection	1. temp within normal range 2. WBC within normal range 3. lungs clear 4. negative sputum culture 5. negative urine culture 6. urine clear many others.....	1. monitor for clinical manifestations of infection: inc. temp, adventitious breath sounds, pain on urination, colored sputum.... 2. monitor labs and report abnormal values 3. implement measures to prevent pneumonia (specify)... 4. implement measures to prevent urinary tract infection (specify)...
#4	High risk for impaired gas exchange	1. Usual skin and mucous membrane color 2. Usual mental status 3. Normal Hg, Hct, ABG	1. Incentive spirometry q 2 hours 2. turn q 2 hours 3. encourage ambulation or chair 4. deep breath and cough q 2 hours 5. maintain oxygen therapy as ordered
#5	High risk for injury: aspiration	1. clear breath sounds 2. normal respiratory rate, rhythm and depth 3. denies dyspnea 4. usual skin color	1. monitor for clinical manifestations of aspiration 2. implement measures to prevent aspiration (specify)...
#6	Self care deficit: feeding	performs feeding activities within physical limitations	1. assess degree of feeding deficit 2. implement measures to facilitate pt. involvement in feeding (specify)...

Reference text: Ulrich SP et al. Nursing care planning guides, 3rd Ed. Saunders.1994

[This ends the Case of Mary Burns]

The Case of Mary Burns, PSE
Script

History/Assessment Data: This is a listing of data to feed students based on their questions in Task #2. They may or may not ask for all of these data in the time you have available. Therefore, having them prioritize is essential. Extra boxes have been left in table for you to fill in other data as you wish.

Parameter	Requested	Data
ECG		Atrial fibrillation
Vital Sign		BP = 90/60, HR = 110, RR = 28, T = 101.5 oral
Cultures		Urine and sputum = negative
Electrolytes, Glucose		$K+ = 4.0$, $Na^+ = 135$, Glucose =170
CBC		Hg = 10.8, Hct = 32%, RBC = 3.5, WBC = 18,000
Neurologic status		GCS = 14, Disoriented to time and place. C/O numbness and tingling
Apparent state of health		Obese. Ht. = 5'3". Usual weight = 190#. Current draining 80 cc/hr
IV Fluids		D5 NS with 20mEq KCL at 75cc/hr per intermittent infusion port
Intake/Output		I = 2000. O = 1500. Urinary catheter is current draining 80cc/hr
Renal function		BUN = 4. serum creatinine = 0.3
Albumin level		2.0 g/dl
Medications		Nifedipine 10mg (SL) TID. Dilantin 100 mg IVPB TID. Decadron 2mg PO TID. HCTZ 5mg PO TID
Activity Status		Up in chair with assistance BID
Diet		Sustacal per enteric feeding tube at 50cc/hr. 10cc residual noted
Past Medical History		Hypertension, coronary artery disease
Chest x-ray		Consistent with atelectasis with small infiltrate LLL
Bowel status		+ bowel sounds in all 4 quads
Heart Sounds		S1 and S2. No murmur
Lung sounds		decreased breath sounds LLF with left > right
Skin & mucous membranes		Skin is warm and clammy. 3+ pedal edema bilaterally. 2+ ascites. Upper extremities. 2+ edema. Reddened area approx. 2 cm in diameter on sacral region
Liver enzymes		within normal limits
Serum Osmolality		310 mOsm
Other:		

PART VI

METABOLISM

Part VI. Table of Contents

PART VI. METABOLISM

Take Home Cases (THC)

Metabolic Responses (Module 20)   165
Altered Immune Function (Module 21)   176
Acute Hepatic Dysfunction (Module 23)   187
Acute Glucose Metabolism (Module 24)   195
Acute Renal Dysfunction (Module 26)   205

Case Studies / Exercise

The Diabetic Crises Cases   213
The Immunocompetence Cases   225
The Case of Joan T.   237
The Case of C.R. Cramer (see also PSE version)   242
The Case of Bob White   252

Problem Solving Exercises (PSE)

The Case of C.R. Cramer (see also Case Study version)   260

Clinical Foci

Endocrine Problems   265
Acute GI Problems   268

Take Home Case
Module 20: Metabolic Responses

Student Name: _____ Date: _____

DIRECTIONS:
        In narrative form, complete the following questions or statements based on the Module reading assignment. To better comprehend this material, it is best to answer the items in your own words rather than copying answers from the text. By doing so, you can evaluate what you actually understand.

READING ASSIGNMENT: *High Acuity Nursing, 2ⁿᵈ ed.* -- Module 20: Metabolic Responses
****
Scenario: Patty T., 23 years old, was in a motorcycle accident in which she sustained multiple trauma. She has been in the hospital for two weeks. Prior to her accident, she had been in excellent health, with no chronic health problems.

SECTION ONE: Metabolism

1. Briefly explain the difference between anabolism and catabolism:

    Do you think Patty is in a state of anabolism or catabolism? Why?

2. The body turns to anaerobic metabolism when there is an inadequate supply of _____. During

    anaerobic metabolism, most body cells use _____ _____ as their source of energy. Levels of

    this substance can be monitored to monitor anaerobic metabolism.

3. Energy is measured in units called _____. The majority of energy needed by the body is used

    to maintain _____ _____ across cell membranes.

SECTION TWO: Nutrition In The High Acuity Patient

During the healing process, Patty has increased needs for macronutrients as well as micronutrients.
---

4. In the space provided, list the macronutrients and describe as indicated:

Macronutrient	Basic Units	Primary Functions

5. Patty's GI status is very important to monitor. Briefly explain the immune functions of the gut:

6. Why is Patty's gut susceptible to ischemic problems?

7. Explain the concept: *bacterial translocation*:

SECTION THREE: Nutritional And Metabolic Assessment

Patty is losing weight. She is having nutrition related testing performed.

8. In the table provided, describe the laboratory data that is commonly used to measure nutritional status:

Test	Normal Values	Half-Life / Significance	Status Being Measured	Potential Sources of Abnormal Values
Albumin	3.5-5.5 g/dL			
Prealbumin	15.7-29.6 mg/mL			
Transferrin	250-300 mg/dL			
Nitrogen Balance	Nitrogen in = nitrogen out			

9. The nurse decides to calculate Patty's Total Lymphocyte Count (TLC). Patty's latest WBC count was 15,000 and her Lymphs were 15%. Calculate her lymphocyte and explain the significance.

10. Why might the physician or nutrition support team want to measure Patty's oxygen consumption and energy expenditure? What is the relationship of oxygen consumption to energy expenditure?

11. What are common causes of increased oxygen consumption and energy expenditure?

What nursing interventions can be performed to decrease oxygen consumption and energy expenditure?

13. Examine Table 20-5: Harris-Benedict Equation and Stress Factors. What three clinical conditions have the highest stress factors? What might be the reasons for this?

SECTION FOUR: Metabolic Alterations In The High Acuity Patient

14. Differentiate marasmus from kwashiorkor types of starvation.

15. Differentiate between the clinical manifestations associated with marasmus and kwashiokor, in high acuity patients

Starvation Type	Common Causes	Associated Clinical Manifestations
Marasmus		
Kwashiorkor		

Both condition are referred to as _____ malnutrition.

16. Under what circumstances do patients, such as Patty, develop starvation?

17. During prolonged periods of starvation, after about two weeks, the body turns to _____ as the major fuel source.

Ebb Vs. Flow Phases of the Metabolic Stress Response

18. During the first 24 hours following her injury, Patty's systemic circulation was probably unchanged or slightly _____. This may be accompanied by a body temperature that is <u>increased / decreased</u> (circle one). This is accompanied by alterations in _____ and _____. This period is called the _____ phase of the metabolic stress response. During this phase, her metabolic rate is _____ and her serum glucose level will be _____.

19. The second phase of the metabolic stress response is the _____ phase. It begins 24 to 36 post insult and lasts 5 to 10 days or longer (until wounds have healed). The 3 characteristics of this phase are _____, and _____. Clinical findings typical of this phase are: _____, _____, _____, and _____.

20. <u>True / False</u> (circle one) During the metabolic stress response, Patty's hyperglycemia is effectively controlled using insulin.

21. Briefly consider (in writing) how the metabolic changes that occur with starvation and those associated with hypermetabolism work against each other.

SECTION FIVE: Nutritional Alterations In Specific Disease States

22. What is the relationship between dysfunction of the following organs and nutritional alterations? This relationship can be a cause or, in some cases, it can be an effect (as in pulmonary failure).

Body System	Altered Nutrition/Metabolic Status
Liver Failure	
Pulmonary Failure	
Acute Renal Failure	
Chronic Renal Failure	

Body System	Altered Nutrition/Metabolic Status
Cardiac Failure	
Gut Failure	
Burns	
Acute Head Injury	

SECTION SIX: Methods Of Enteral Nutrition

23. Assuming Patty cannot take in food PO, what three criteria will be used to help determine whether she should receive enteric feedings?

> **It is decided that Patty will receive enteral feedings as long as no contraindications are present.**

24. List two contraindications to enteral feeding:

> *Patty develops a complication of enteral nutrition.*

25. The small bore feeding tube becomes occluded. In your own words, describe two methods for unplugging the tube:

26. What are possible causes of diarrhea in patients receiving enteral nutrition?

SECTION SEVEN: Methods of Total Parenteral Nutrition

> Patty's bowel function has become minimal. It is decided to trickle in small quantities of tube feeding but to initiate TPN as the primary mode of nutritional support.

28. TPN is highly concentrated and needs to run through a _____ vein. The vein of choice is the _____.

29. Indications for TPN use are:

30. List two clinical signs and symptoms of catheter related sepsis, a complication of TPN therapy.

31. TPN can affect kidney function when too much protein is administered, causing what two problems?
     A.
     B.

Congratulations, you have completed this Take Home Case

Take Home Case
Module 20: Metabolic Responses
Instructor Guide

DIRECTIONS:
In narrative form, complete the following questions or statements based on the Module reading assignment. To better comprehend this material, it is best to answer the items in your own words rather than copying answers from the text. By doing so, you can evaluate what you actually understand.

READING ASSIGNMENT: *High Acuity Nursing, 2nd ed.* -- Module 20: Metabolic Responses
****
Scenario: Patty T., 23 years old, was in a motorcycle accident in which sustained multiple trauma. She has been in the hospital for two weeks. Prior to her accident, she had been in excellent health, with no chronic health problems.

SECTION ONE: Metabolism

1. Briefly explain the difference between anabolism and catabolism:
   Anabolism is a constructive process that contributes to tissue building. It requires energy.
   Catabolism is a destructive process that contributes to tissue breakdown. It provides energy.

   Do you think Patty is in a state of anabolism or catabolism? Why?
   She is most likely in a state of catabolism due to the high level of traumatic stress. Her multiple trauma will require extensive healing, which will tax her nutrition status.

2. The body turns to anaerobic metabolism when there is an inadequate supply of __*oxygen*__. During anaerobic metabolism, most body cells use _*lactic*_ _*acid*__ as their source of energy. Levels of this substance can be monitored to monitor anaerobic metabolism.

3. Energy is measured in units called ___*calories*_. The majority of energy needed by the body is used to maintain _*ion*__ _*gradients*_ across cell membranes.

SECTION TWO: Nutrition In The High Acuity Patient

During the healing process, Patty has increased needs for macronutrients as well as micronutrients.
---

4. In the space provided, list the macronutrients and describe as indicated:

Macronutrient	Basic Units	Primary Functions
Carbohydrates	sugars, starches	Primary source of energy for most tissues
Proteins	amino acids	Essential for formation & maintenance of all cells. Contribute to structure of muscle, organs, antibodies, enzymes, hormones.
Lipids (fats)	fatty acids	Contribute to cell membrane structure. Primary source of fuel reserve

5. Patty's GI status is very important to monitor. Briefly explain the immune functions of the gut:
   The submucosa contains lymph system. The mucosa (innermost) layer is the site of immune activities. It forms a barrier between GI contents and the sterile abdominal contents.

6. Why is Patty's gut susceptible to ischemic problems?

The mucosal cells of the gut have a high energy requirement, thus are dependent on a steady supply of nutrients and oxygen to maintain proper functioning. It is very susceptible to hypoxia and diminished tissue perfusion.

7. Explain how the concept: *bacterial translocation*:
Tissue hypoxia in the gut interrupts the barrier defense mechanism, allowing microbes to migrate out of the gut into the sterile surrounding tissues (blood vessels, lymphatics, and/or peritoneal cavity). It is considered to be a major source of multisystem organ dysfunction (MODS).

SECTION THREE: Nutritional And Metabolic Assessment

Patty is losing weight. She is having nutrition related testing performed.

8. In the table provided, describe the laboratory data that is commonly used to measure nutritional status:

Test	Normal Values	Half-Life / Significance	Status Being Measured	Potential Sources of Abnormal Values
Albumin	3.5-5.5 g/dL	*20 days- not good indicator of <u>acute</u> malnutrition*	*Visceral protein status*	*Malnutrition; liver disease, renal disease; fluid resuscitation (dilutional effect)*
Prealbumin	15.7-29.6 mg/mL	*24 - 48 hours - good indicator of current nutrition status*	*Visceral protein status*	*Malnutrition; fluid resuscitation (dilutional effect); dehydration*
Transferrin	250-300 mg/dL	*8-10 days; better than albumin but not as good as prealbumin for measuring acute changes*	*Visceral protein status*	*Malnutrition; iron deficiency anemia*
Nitrogen Balance	Nitrogen in = nitrogen out	*N/A*	*Protein status*	*Inadequate protein intake; stress; protein catabolism*

9. The nurse decides to calculate Patty's Total Lymphocyte Count (TLC). Patty's latest WBC count was 15,000 and her Lymphs were 15%. Calculate her lymphocyte and explain the significance.
Formula = TLC = WBC X % lymphs ÷ 100. (15,000 X 15) ÷ 100 = 2250. This level falls within the normal range. Its significance is that her immune function is adequate at this time.

10. Why might the physician or nutrition support team want to measure Patty's oxygen consumption and energy expenditure? What is the relationship of oxygen consumption to energy expenditure?
To measure her metabolic state. They have a direct relationship -- As oxygen consumption goes up, so does energy expenditure.

11. What are common causes of increased oxygen consumption and energy expenditure?
Fever, shivering, pain, increases in environmental temperature, physical activity

What nursing interventions can be performed to decrease oxygen consumption and energy expenditure?
Fever and chills are usually controlled through drug therapy, such as acetaminophen. Tepid sponge baths, ice packs, and cooling blankets are also sometimes used. Room temperature is usually kept cool with the exception of burn injury. Physical activities / stimulation may be

controlled and/or limited to some degree. Nursing interventions may be spaced out to decrease length of time for a single physical exertion episode. Research continues in this area.

13. Examine Table 20-5: Harris-Benedict Equation and Stress Factors. What three clinical conditions have the highest stress factors? What might be the reasons for this?
    Burn injury before skin grafting, sepsis (normotensive), and major surgery are the three highest. All are extremely hypermetabolic processes -- all are massive physiologic insults. Burned tissue loses heat, fluid, and nutrients at exceptionally high rates. Sepsis is a systemic insult that taxes multiple body systems. Major surgery requires increased metabolic processes to facilitate healing.

SECTION FOUR: Metabolic Alterations In The High Acuity Patient

14. Differentiate marasmus from kwashiorkor types of starvation.
    Marasmus results from inadequate intake of protein and calories. Somatic proteins are inadequate. It is associated with generalized body wasting. Kwashiorkor results from adequate intake of carbohydrates but inadequate protein intake. Visceral proteins are inadequate. It is associated with sparing of muscle but loss of albumin and immunoglobulins.

15. Differentiate between the clinical manifestations associated with marasmus and kwashiokor, in high acuity patients.

Starvation Type	Common Causes	Associated Clinical Manifestations
Marasmus	Alt. GI function; prolonged anorexia. Can lead to kwashiorkor	Skeletal muscle wasting; loss of fat stores; decreased activity tolerance; weight loss
Kwashiorkor	As a continuation/ worsening of marasmus – particularly accompanied by new insult such as surgery, injury, or infection	Diminished immune system function (particularly antibodies); edema; decreased serum albumin levels

Both condition are referred to as ___*protein-energy*_ malnutrition.

16. Under what circumstances do patients, such as Patty, develop starvation?
    High acuity patient can be easily starved by failure to give adequate nutritional support. When patients are hypermetabolic due to trauma, stress, infection, etc., they require more nutrients to meet the increased level of oxygen consumption and energy expenditure. Patients may be kept NPO for prolonged periods of time, or if nutrients are given, they may not be sufficient to meet the individual needs of the stress patient.

17. During prolonged periods of starvation, after about two weeks, the body turns to _*fat*__ as the major fuel source.

Ebb Vs. Flow Phases of the Metabolic Stress Response

18. During the first 24 hours following her injury, Patty's systemic circulation was probably unchanged or slightly *decreased*. This may be accompanied by a body temperature that is increased / *decreased* (circle one). This is accompanied by alterations in _*carbohydrate*_ and __lipid_ *metabolism*__. This period is called the __*ebb*__ phase of the metabolic stress response. During this phase, her metabolic rate is *decreased* and her serum glucose level will be _*hyperglycemic*_.

19. The second phase of the metabolic stress response is the _flow_ phase. It begins 24 to 36 post insult and lasts 5 to 10 days or longer (until wounds have healed). The 3 characteristics of this phase are _**hypermetabolism**_, and _**hypercatabolism**_. Clinical findings typical of this phase are: __*tachycardia*_, __*tachypnea*__, __*increased cardiac output*_, and __*fever*__.

20. True / _**False**_ (circle one) During the metabolic stress response, Patty's hyperglycemia is effectively controlled using insulin.

21. Briefly consider (in writing) how the metabolic changes that occur with starvation and those associated with hypermetabolism, work against each other.

    The effects of starvation cause metabolism to slow down to conserve energy, sparing proteins in favor of fat as the primary source of energy. Starvation, however, decreases protein synthesis, thus healing is significantly reduced. Hypermetabolism causes a significant increase in metabolic processes, consuming large amounts of energy, requiring the body to provide the energy through secondary resources of protein and fat catabolism. Therefore, while starvation conserves and reduces, hypermetabolism significantly increases demands.

SECTION FIVE: Nutritional Alterations In Specific Disease States

22. What is the relationship between dysfunction of the following organs and nutritional alterations? This relationship can be a cause or, in some cases, it can be an effect (as in pulmonary failure).

Body System	*Altered Nutrition/Metabolic Status*
Liver Failure	*When liver function is significantly decreased, the it can have the following effects: Hypercatabolism. Release of aromatic amino acids (AAA) into CNS may contribute to hepatic encephalopathy; decreased ability to use fat for energy; hyperglycemia; hyponatremia.*
Pulmonary Failure	*Pulmonary failure can result from malnutrition since the respiratory muscles may be catabolized. If malnutrition related edema is severe, it can precipitate pulmonary edema which can alter gas exchange. Malnutrition also decreases immune function which increases the risk of pneumonia.*
Acute Renal Failure	*Metabolic waste products can build up. Associated nutritional alterations include hypercatabolism, hypermetabolism, electrolyte and trace element abnormalities, and fluid retention.*
Chronic Renal Failure	*Patients in chronic renal failure develop anorexia, nausea and delayed gastric emptying secondary to uremia. Weight loss and loss of lean body mass.*
Cardiac Failure	*Cardiac failure can result from severe protein-energy malnutrition since the heart muscle is not spared from muscle wasting associated with malnutrition. Low levels of many electrolytes impair cardiac contractility. Thiamine deficiency can vasodilate peripheral blood vessels.*
Gut Failure	*If tissue perfusion to the gut is compromised, gut permeability increases and bacterial translocation can result.*
Burns	*Major burn injury significantly increases energy, protein, fluid needs. The level of hypermetabolic response depends on the severity of the burn.*
Acute Head Injury	*Causes extreme hypermetabolic and hypercatabolic processes. The level of hypermetabolism is inversely proportional to the Glasgow Coma Score. The brain requires highest O_2 consumption of all organs.*

SECTION SIX: Methods Of Enteral Nutrition

22. Assuming Patty cannot take in food PO, what three criteria will be used to help determine whether she should receive enteric feedings?

    The decision will be made on the basis of his GI function, baseline nutritional status, and present catabolic state & possible duration.

It is decided that Patty will receive enteral feedings as long as no contraindications are present.
---

23. List two contraindications to enteral feeding:

    Contraindications to enteral feeding include any two of the following: 1) adynamic ileum; 2) intractable vomiting; 3) presence of proximal high output enterocutaneous fistula; 4) bowel needs to rest; 5) active GI bleeding.

Patty develops a complication of enteral nutrition.
---

24. The small bore feeding tube becomes occluded. In your own words, describe two methods for unplugging the tube:

    The nurse may have any of the following options to try to open the occluded tube: 1) irrigate the tube with 30 - 50 mL of warm water every 4 hours, following medications, and following checking residuals. 2) alternate positive and negative pressure with a syringe to dislodge the occlusion; 3) use meat tenderizer, colas or pancrease/HCO_3.

25. What are possible causes of diarrhea in patients receiving enteral nutrition?

    Antibiotics may alter intestinal flora causing bacterial overgrowth: Clostridium difficile infection and pseudomembranous colitis.

SECTION SEVEN: Methods of Total Parenteral Nutrition

Patty's bowel function has become minimal. It is decided to trickle in small quantities of tube feeding but to initiate TPN as the primary mode of nutritional support.
---

26. TPN is highly concentrated and needs to run through a __*central*__ vein. The vein of choice is the __*subclavian*__.

27. Indications for TPN use are:

    When adequate nutrition cannot be delivered via GI tract because: 1) Bowel must rest (e.g., Crohn's disease, acute pancreatitis); 2) A disruption in GI tract (e.g., bowel obstruction).

28. List two clinical signs and symptoms of catheter related sepsis, a complication of TPN therapy.

    The clinical signs and symptoms of CRS can include any two of the following: bacteremia/ septicemia/septic shock; leukocytosis; sudden temperature elevation that should reduce on catheter removal; sudden glucose intolerance up to 12 hours prior to temperature elevation; or erythema, swelling, tenderness, purulent drainage at the catheter entry site.

29. TPN can affect kidney function when too much protein is administered, causing what two problems?

    A. *Elevated BUN*
    B. *signs of dehydration*

Take Home Case
Module 21: Altered Immune Function

STUDENT NAME: _____. DATE: _____.

DIRECTIONS:

      In narrative form, complete the following questions or statements based on the Module reading assignment. To better comprehend this material, it is best to answer the items in your own words rather than copying answers from the text. By doing so, you can evaluate what you actually understand.

READING ASSIGNMENT: *High Acuity Nursing, 2nd ed.* -- Module 21: Altered Immune Function.
****

SITUATION: *Diana Cheung was admitted to the hospital 5 days ago with a diagnosis of exacerbation of her leukemia. Diana is currently undergoing chemotherapy.*

SECTION ONE: Role of the Immune System in Body Defense

1. List the major immune related functions of the following primary organs of Diana's immune system:

        ORGAN   **PRIMARY IMMUNE FUNCTIONS**

    1. Thymus

    2. Lymph System

    3. Spleen

SECTION TWO: Characteristics of the Immune System

2. At birth, Diana had what type of immunity?

3. As a child, Diana was vaccinated against polio. This is an example of _____ immunity.

4. At one time, Diana also had received gamma globulin when she was exposed to hepatitis at work. Receiving gamma globulin is an example of _____ immunity.

5. Diana has an antibody titer drawn. How is adequate immunity established, using this test?

SECTION THREE: Antigens and Antigen-Antibody Response

6. Define: pathogenic antigen --

7. An example of a nonpathogenic antigen is a _____.

8. Proteins found on the cell surface that help distinguish self from non-self are called:

9. Explain the significance of tumor-associated antigens:

10. A specific immune response involves:

Diana's disease involves dysfunctional lymphocytes.

SECTION FOUR: Cells of the Immune Response

11. In the space provided, state the function of each of the following:

Type of Cell	**Function**
T-Lymphocytes (T cells)	
Killer T cells	
Helper T cells	
B Lymphocytes	
Macrophage	
Cytokines (e.g., IL, TNF)	

12. Briefly explain the term CD marker:

SECTION FIVE: Mechanisms of Immunity

13. **Humoral** immunity involves _____ lymphocyte activity while **cell-mediated** immunity involves _____ lymphocyte activity.

14. Diana's immunoglobulins are made up of _____. They are also called _____. The most common class of immunoglobulin is _____ and it protects newborns.

15. IgA is predominately found where?

15. A secondary humoral response occurs when:

16. If Diana receives a vaccination, you would expect her antibody titer level to increase / decrease (circle one).

17. A vaccination is an example of which type of immune response?

18. Briefly explain chemotaxis:

19. Interferons (INFs) serve what functions?

SECTION SIX: Pathogenesis of Hypersensivity and Autoimmunity

20. If Diana developed anaphylaxis, in what way is histamine involved in this extreme form of hypersensitivity reaction?

What are the typical clinical findings associated with anaphylaxis and what is the general cause of these findings?

Body System	Clinical Findings	Cause
Cardiovascular		
Respiratory		
Cutaneous		
Gastrointestinal		

> **Diana develops a transfusion reaction while receiving a unit of blood.**

20. Diana's transfusion reaction is due to a Type _____ response, which is also called a _____ _____.
    This type of reaction is particularly destructive to _____.

This ends the Case of Diana

21. When a person develops an autoimmune disease, what is the basic problem?

SECTION SEVEN: Systemic Lupus Erythematosus: A Manifestation of Autoimmunity

Scenario:
Barbara Martin is a 26 year old nursing student. Barbara was seen by her family physician with the following physical complaints: fatigue, fevers, and arthritic-type joint pain, which is often severe. Labs are drawn on Barbara. She is diagnosed with systemic lupus erythematosus (SLE).
****

22. Barbara's SLE is believed to be a type _III_ response. It is characterized by _____

    _____ deposits in the epithelial lining of _____ _____ and tissue surfaces.

23. Briefly describe the pathologic events associated with SLE that lead to impaired organ function:

24. Who is at particular risk for development of SLE?

25. Barbara's SLE is not an organ-nonspecific disease. List the organs that are most commonly attacked:

26. Although the clinical findings associated with SLE depend on which organs are involved, what symptoms do most SLE patients experience?

27. Diagnosing Barbara's SLE can be difficult. Match the test with the appropriate description. (Some tests may have more than one description)

Test	*Description*
_____ LE cell test	A. Absence of this antibody strongly suggests SLE is not present
_____ Antinuclear antibody (ANA)	B. Quite specific to SLE
_____ Anti-DNA antibodies	C. Screening test; not specific for SLE
_____ Anti-SM antibodies	D. Levels frequently parallel the disease
	E. Early, non-specific test; has been largely replaced

28. Barbara's regular treatment will typically include:

If she develops uncontrolled lupus, called a "flare", what types of drug therapy is she likely to have ordered?

This Ends the Case of Barbara Martin

SECTION EIGHT: HIV Disease: A Manifestation of Immunodeficiency

29. The term "primary immunodeficiency" refers to:

30. Secondary immunodeficiencies most commonly result from what 3 things?

31. What does the term "acquired immunodeficiency" refer to?

32. The human immunodeficiency virus (HIV) selectively invades and infects the _____ cells but does not seem to affect the _____ cells.

33. HIV is a retrovirus. What makes a retrovirus different from other viruses?

35. The laboratory test that is 95 to 99% accurate at identifying the presence of HIV antibody is the:

36. Confirmation of a diagnosis of HIV infection requires what test combination?

37. True / False (circle one). The meaning of the term HIV is the same as AIDS.

38. The 1993 revised AIDS definition includes what 5 criteria?
    a)

    b)

    c)

    d)

    e)

SECTION NINE: Aging, Malnutrition, Stress, Trauma, and the Immue System

39. Malnutrition particularly affects which type of lymphocytes?

40. Stress affects the immune system due to increased production of _____, which inhibits _____ and _____, resulting in _____ cell response

SECTION TEN: Care of the Immunocompromised Patient

We now return to the Case of Diana Cheung: Diana was admitted to the hospital 5 days ago with a diagnosis of exacerbation of her leukemia. She is currently undergoing chemotherapy. Her laboratory tests show that she is becoming immunocompromised.

41. When performing a physical assessment on an immunocompromised patient, such as Diana, the nurse should focus on assessing for evidence of _____.

42. The WBC with differential cell count is a valuable test for assessing level of immunocompetence.. Complete the table below as directed:

Test	Normal Range (in % of total WBC)	Major Function	Trend # ($\Uparrow$ or $\Downarrow$); Appropriate Term # Immunodeficient conditions
WBC (leukocytes)	4,500 to 10,000 μL		
Neutrophils	50 - 70%		

Test	Normal Range (in % of total WBC)	Major Function	Trend [#] (⇑ or ⇓); Appropriate Term [#] Immunodeficient conditions
Lymphocytes	25 - 35%		
Monocytes	4-6%		

43. Two major goals for managing Diana's care are to reestablish immunocompetence, and prevent/treat complications. Consider what aspect of these goals can be dealt with by the nurse.

44. Explain in what ways clinical findings associated with infection in the neutropenic patient differs from patients with normal neutrophil counts:

Take Home Case
Module 21: Altered Immune Function
Instructor Guide

DIRECTIONS
      In narrative form, complete the following questions or statements based on the Module reading assignment. To better comprehend this material, it is best to answer the items in your own words rather than copying answers from the text. By doing so, you can evaluate what you actually understand.

Required Reading Assignment: *High Acuity Nursing, 2ⁿᵈ ed.* -- Module 21: Altered Immune Function
****

SITUATION: *Diana Cheung was admitted to the hospital 5 days ago with a diagnosis of exacerbation of her leukemia. Diana is currently undergoing chemotherapy.*

SECTION ONE: Role of the Immune System in Body Defense

1. List the major immune related functions of the following primary organs of Diana's immune system:

ORGAN	PRIMARY IMMUNE FUNCTIONS
1. Thymus	*differentiates lymphocytes into types of T cells*
2. Lymph System	*filtering system for foreign materials; reservoir for T & B cells*
3. Spleen	*reservoir for B cells*

SECTION TWO: Characteristics of the Immune System

2. At birth, Diana had what type of immunity? *Natural*

3. As a child, Diana was vaccinated against polio. This is an example of __*active*__ immunity.

4. At one time, Diana also had received gamma globulin when she was exposed to hepatitis at work. Receiving gamma globulin is an example of __*passive*__ immunity.

5. Diana has an antibody titer drawn. How is adequate immunity established, using this test?
      Her titer will be compared to a standard antibody level that is thought to guarantee immunity. If her level is lower than the standard, she may require reimmunization.

SECTION THREE: Antigens and Antigen-Antibody Response

6. Define: pathogenic antigen -- *a foreign material capable of producing disease.*

7. An example of a nonpathogenic antigen is a __*transplanted organ*__.

8. Proteins found on the cell surface that help distinguish self from non-self are called __*histocompatibility antigens (or HLA)*__.

9. Explain the significance of tumor-associated antigens:
      Elevated levels of certain antigens can be helpful in detecting potentially abnormal cells and tracking progression of disease or regression of disease following treatment.

10. A specific immune response involves: *1) recognition of a particular antigen, and 2) production and action of a specific antibody.*

> **Diana's disease involves dysfunctional lymphocytes.**

SECTION FOUR: Cells of the Immune Response

11. In the space provided, state the function of each of the following:

Type of Cell	Function
T-Lymphocytes (T cells)	*Responsible for cell mediated immunity*
Killer T cells	*Attack & destroy antigens*
Helper T cells	*Enhance action of B cells*
B Lymphocytes	*Antibody production*
Macrophage	*Phagocytosis; processes the antigen*
Cytokines (e.g., IL, TNF)	***Immune mediators; chemical messengers***

12. Briefly explain the term CD marker:
    The initials, CD, stand for "clusters of differentiation". The clusters are surface antigens located on T cells. For example, helper T cells have a CD4 marker. HIV attacks cells with the CD4 marker.

SECTION FIVE: Mechanisms of Immunity

13. Humoral immunity involves __*B cell*__ lymphocyte activity while cell-mediated immunity involves __*T cell*__ lymphocyte activity.

14. Diana's Immunoglobulins are made up of ____*plasma proteins*___. They are also called _____*antibodies*____. The most common class of immunoglobulin is __*IgG*__ and it protects newborns.

15. IgA is predominately found where?
    body secretions (saliva, nasal & resp. secretions, breast milk).

15. A secondary humoral response occurs when: ***there is a subsequent exposure to the same antigen.***

16. If Diana receives a vaccination, you would expect her antibody titer level to *increase* / decrease (circle one)

17. A vaccination is an example of which type of immune response? ***humoral secondary response***

18. Briefly explain chemotaxis:
    The chemical attraction of phagocytic cells to antigens and engulfing of antigens for purposes of destruction or neutralization.

19. Interferons (INFs) serve what functions?
    Important defense mechanism against viruses and other intracellular pathogens. Inhibit synthesis of viral protein without harming the host's protein synthesis. Strong activator of macrophage activity.

SECTION SIX: Pathogenesis of Hypersensivity and Autoimmunity

20. If Diana developed anaphylaxis, in what way is histamine involved in this extreme form of hypersensitivity reaction?
    Anaphylaxis is a type 1 response. Mast cells release histamine and other substances. Histamine is a power vasodilator. When it is released, capillaries become more permeable, causing leaking; smooth muscle contracts; and constriction of the bronchi.

    What are the typical clinical findings associated with anaphylaxis and what is the general cause of these findings?

Body System	Clinical Findings	Cause
Cardiovascular	*Profound hypotension, decreased cardiac output, myocardial ischemia*	*vasodilation, increased capillary permeability*
Respiratory	*Bronchoconstriction*	*Smooth muscle contraction, bronchial constriction*
Cutaneous	*Urticaria (hives)*	*IgE-mast cell interaction in which receptors in cutaneous blood vessels cause redness & swelling*
Gastrointestinal	*Crampy pain, nausea, diarrhea*	*Smooth muscle contraction & edema of GI mucosa*

> **Diana develops a transfusion reaction while receiving a unit of blood.**

20. Diana's transfusion reaction is due to a Type __*II*___ response, which is also called a __*cytotoxic*__ __*reaction*__. This type of reaction is particularly destructive to __*RBCs*__.

This ends the Case of Diana

21. When a person develops an autoimmune disease, what is basic problem?
    The body recognizes "self" as foreign and initiates a destructive response.

SECTION SEVEN: Systemic Lupus Erythematosus: A Manifestation of Autoimmunity
Scenario:
    Barbara Martin is a 26 year old nursing student. Barbara was seen by her family physician with the following physical complaints: fatigue, fevers, and arthritic-type joint pain, which is often severe. Labs are drawn on Barbara. She is diagnosed with systemic lupus erythematosus (SLE).
****

22. Barbara's SLE is believed to be a type _III_ response. It is characterized by _*antigen-antibody*_ ___*complex*___ deposits in the epithelial lining of _*blood*_ _*vessels*_ and tissue surfaces.

23. Briefly describe the pathologic events associated with SLE that lead to impaired organ function:
    Antigen-antibody complex deposits cause occlusion and inflammation which causes local damage, including edema, hemorrhage, clotting, neutrophil accumulation. Vessel occlusions lead to death of tissue and scar formation.

24. Who is at particular risk for development of SLE?
    Women during childbearing years; higher incidence in African Americans and Asians; exposure to ultra violet light; certain chemicals (e.g., procainamide, hair dyes, hydralazine); estrogen

25. Barbara's SLE is not an organ-nonspecific disease. List the organs that are most commonly attacked:
    Kidneys, brain, heart, lungs, connective tissues, spleen

26. Although the clinical findings associated with SLE depend on which organs are involved, what symptoms to most SLE patients experience?
    Malaise, fatigue, fever, ski manifestations (rashes and patches), joint pain

27. Diagnosing Barbara's SLE can be difficult. Match the test with the appropriate description. (Some tests may have more than one description)

Test	*Description*
__E__ LE cell test	A. Absence of this antibody strongly suggests SLE is not present
_A,C_ Antinuclear antibody (ANA)	B. Quite specific to SLE
_B,D_ Anti-DNA antibodies	C. Screening test; not specific for SLE
_B,D_ Anti-SM antibodies	D. Levels frequently parallel the disease
	E. Early, non-specific test; has been largely replaced

28. Barbara's regular treatment will typically include:
    Nonsteroidal antiinflammatory drugs (NSAID), antimalarial drugs. If symptoms become severe, high-dose corticosteroids.

    If she develops uncontrolled lupus, called a "flare", what types of drug therapy is she likely to have ordered? *azathioprine (Imuran), cyclophosphamide (Cytoxan), or methotrexate*

This Ends the Case of Barbara Martin

SECTION EIGHT: HIV Disease: A Manifestation of Immunodeficiency

29. The term "primary immunodeficiency" refers to: *a state of deficiency of the immune system that is caused by a genetic anomaly of the immune system.*

30. Secondary immunodeficiencies most commonly result from what 3 things?
    1) other primary diseases (e.g., Hodgkin's disease), 2) drug therapy (e.g., corticosteroid therapy), and 3) irradiation therapy

31. What does the term "acquired immunodeficiency" refer to?
    immunodeficiency caused by a direct attack on the immune system by pathogens

32. The human immunodeficiency virus (HIV) selectively invades and infects the __T__ cells but does not seem to affect the __C__ cells.

33. HIV is a retrovirus. What makes a retrovirus different from other viruses?
    A retrovirus carries genetic information in RNA rather than in DNA.

35. The laboratory test that is 95 to 99% accurate at identifying the presence of HIV antibody is the:
    enzyme-linked immunosorbent assay (ELISA)

36. Confirmation of a diagnosis of HIV infection requires what test combination?
    2 positive ELISAs and a positive Western blot test

37. True / *False* (circle one). The meaning of the term HIV is the same as AIDS.

38. The 1993 revised AIDS definition includes what 5 criteria?
    a) *seropositive HIV infection*
    b) *CD4 count less than 200/µL*
    c) *recurrent pneumonia (e.g., Pneumocystis carinii)*
    d) *tuberculosis*
    e) *invasive cervical cancer*

SECTION NINE: Aging, Malnutrition, Stress, Trauma, and the Immune System

39. Malnutrition particularly affects which type of lymphocytes? *T cells*

40. Stress affects the immune system due to increased production of *__cortisol__*, which inhibits *__interleukin I__* and *__interleukin II__*, resulting in *__decreased__* T cell response

SECTION TEN: Care of the Immunocompromised Patient

> **We now return to the Case of Diana Cheung:** Diana was admitted to the hospital 5 days ago with a diagnosis of exacerbation of her leukemia. She is currently undergoing chemotherapy. Her laboratory tests show that she is becoming immunocompromised.

41. When performing a physical assessment on an immunocompromised patient, such as Diana, the nurse should focus on assessing for evidence of ____*infection*____.

42. The WBC with differential cell count is a valuable test for assessing level of immunocompetence. Complete the table below as directed:

Test	Normal Range (in % of total WBC)	Major Function	Trend # ($\Uparrow$ or $\Downarrow$); Appropriate Term # Immunodeficient conditions
WBC (leukocytes)	4,500 to 10,000 µL	*Body defense*	$\Downarrow$; *leukopenia*
Neutrophils	50 - 70%	*Rapid response phagocytes; travel rapidly to site of injury.*	$\Downarrow$; *neutropenia*
Lymphocytes	25 - 35%	*Longer term protection; respond to viral & chronic infections*	$\Downarrow$; *lymphocytopenia*
Monocytes	4-6%	*Macrophages; slow to respond; very powerful; ingest & destroy large substances*	$\Downarrow$; *monocytopenia*

43. Two major goals for managing Diana's care are to reestablish immunocompetence, and prevent/treat complications. Consider what aspect of these goals can be dealt with by the nurse.
    Many of the interventions to reestablish immunocompetence are medical interventions. The nurse taking care of an immunocompromised patient spends much of the time assessing for complications and monitoring for the effectiveness of the medical interventions. In addition, the nurse is, in large part, responsible for environmental protection as well as ongoing protection from developing an infection. These activities are crucial to the immunocompromised patient's welfare.

44. Explain in what ways clinical findings associated with infection in the neutropenic patient differs from patients with normal neutrophil counts:
    The severely neutropenic patient will have an alteration in the ability to muster a fever - a fever of 100.5 or above for > 12 hours may be the only sign of infection. Fever is the most important indicator of infection in this patient population – and may be the only distinct early manifestation. The severely neutropenic patient may not be able to form pus – this has important implications on the nurse's usual assessment criteria for infection. A urinary tract infection may not develop cloudy urine. Purulent sputum may not form and adventitious breath sounds may not develop until very late in an infection; an infected wound may not become purulent.

Take Home Case
Module 23: Acute Hepatic Dysfunction

DIRECTIONS:

In narrative form, complete the following questions or statements based on the Module reading assignment. To better comprehend this material, it is best to answer the items in your own words rather than copying answers from the text. By doing so, you can evaluate what you actually understand.

Required Reading: *High Acuity Nursing, 2ⁿᵈ ed.* -- Module 23: Altered Hepatic Dysfunction
****

> **SITUATION: Rachel M., 32 years old, is admitted to the hospital following a suicide attempt in which she consumed a large quantity of acetaminophen.**

SECTION ONE: Anatomy of the Liver

1. The functional unit of the liver is the _____. The purpose of hepatocytes located in the lobules is to secrete the substance _____.

2. Bile is primarily composed of _____ and it is stored in the _____.

3. The term "splanchnic circulation" refers to:

   The liver accepts blood via the _____ vein, from the spleen, intestines, pancreas, and stomach.

   The _____ vein drains blood away from the liver, dumping into the

   _____.

SECTION TWO: Functions of the Liver

5. Examine Table 23-1. Major functions of the liver. If Rachel were to develop congestive heart failure, how would the liver respond?

   What liver related assessments, made by the nurse, would support the presence of CHF?

5. If Rachel had iron deficiency anemia, what role could her dysfunctional liver have played in this problem?

6. Rachel's liver dysfunction has significantly reduced the number of Kupffer's cells. What impact can this have on her outcomes?

SECTION THREE: Evaluation of Liver Function Through Laboratory Tests

> Rachel has liver enzyme and isoenzyme levels drawn.

7. How do enzyme levels reflect liver function?

8. What diagnostic advantages do isoenzymes have over their parent enzymes? Give examples of isoenzymes involved in liver functions.

Rachel has additional laboratory testing done, with the following results: Total bilirubin = 27.3 mg/dL; Serum Albumin = 2.2 g/dL; PT = 14.8 seconds; Ammonia - 42 µg/dL.

---

9. Why do bilirubin levels increase?

10. Rachel's ammonia level is high normal at this point. Where does the ammonia come from?

11. Rachel's serum albumin is low. Consider what you know about the multisystem implications of low albumin. What clinical findings will you monitor her for and why?

SECTION FOUR: Acute Hepatitis

12. True / False (circle one). Acute hepatitis is most commonly caused by a bacterial infection.

Rachel is diagnosed with acute hepatitis secondary to acetaminophen toxicity

---

13. In the space provided, match the description, to the correct type of hepatitis. Some will have several correct responses.

TYPE		DESCRIPTION
_____ Hepatitis A		A. not a complete virus; requires surface antigen of hepatitis
_____ Hepatitis B		B. transmission is via fecal-oral route
_____ Hepatitis C		C. associated with increased risk for chronic liver disease
_____ Hepatitis D		D. transmission is via blood serum or body fluids
_____ Hepatitis E		E. at-risk group is similar to that of H.I.V.
		F. transmission is via contaminated food or water
		G. transmission is via contaminated needles or body fluids

14. Rachel's category of acute hepatitis is "submassive hepatic necrosis". How does this category differ from "classic hepatitis"?

15. If she develops cholestatis hepatitis, what clinical findings will develop?

SECTION FIVE: Acute Hepatic Failure

> **Rachel's condition worsens. She is tentatively diagnosed with acute liver failure.**

16. Rachel's liver failure has most likely resulted from what?

17. Rachel develops hepatic encephalopathy. It is currently being staged. Her current status is as follows: she is lethargic and drowsy. She has slurred speech and she is disoriented. This clinical presentation would place her at what stage of hepatic encephalopathy?

18. As Rachel's carbohydrate metabolism becomes impaired, the nurse can expect increasing hyperglycemia / hypoglycemia (circle one).

SECTION SIX: Complications of Hepatic Dysfunction

19. While she is in liver failure, Rachel is at risk for developing certain complications. In the table below, fill in the major associated clinical findings related to each of the common complications of liver dysfunction.

Complication	Major Associated Clinical Findings
Hepatic encephalopathy	
Portal hypertension	
Esophageal varices	
Ascites	
Hepatorenal syndrome	
Infection	

SECTION SEVEN: Medical Management

20. <u>True / False</u> (circle one). The medical treatment for viral hepatitis is composed of a specific drug regimen.

21. Briefly describe interventions that reduce ammonia toxins.

22. To help protect Rachel from developing GI bleeding, the nurse can anticipate what type of therapy?

23. Although in Rachel's situation bleeding esophageal varices are not likely, if it was believed that she was at risk for.developing them, what general preventive therapy could the nurse anticipate?

SECTION EIGHT: Nursing Implications

24. A major focus of the nursing assessment of the patient with hepatic dysfunction is monitoring for signs and symptoms of _____.

25. During Rachel's latest assessment, the nurse observed involuntary tremors in Rachel's hands. What is the called, and what complication is it associated with?

26. Rachel's skin has become extremely dry and flaky and her skin turgor is poor. These integumentary assessments are caused by:

27. Rachel's breathing pattern is abnormally shallow and rapid. What pathophysiologic events may account for this altered breathing pattern?

28. Rachel is at increased risk for infection. Why is this a potential problem?

You Have Completed This Case

Take Home Case
Module 23: Acute Hepatic Dysfunction
Instructor Guide

DIRECTIONS:
In narrative form, complete the following questions or statements based on the Module reading assignment. To better comprehend this material, it is best to answer the items in your own words rather than copying answers from the text. By doing so, you can evaluate what you actually understand.

Required Reading: *High Acuity Nursing, 2nd ed.* Module 23: Altered Hepatic Dysfunction
****

SITUATION: Rachel M., 32 years old, is admitted to the hospital following a suicide attempt in which she consumed a large quantity of acetaminophen.

SECTION ONE: Anatomy of the Liver

1. The functional unit of the liver is the __*lobule*__. The purpoe of hepatocytes located in the lobules is to secrete the substance __*bile*___.

2. Bile is primarily composed of __*bile salts*__ and it is stored in the ___*gallbladder*____.

3. The term "splanchnic circulation" refers to:
   circulation of the abdominal organs (viscera).

   The liver accepts blood via the __*portal*__ vein, from the spleen, intestines, pancreas, and stomach. The __*hepatic*__ vein drains blood away from the liver, dumping into the __*inferior vena cava*__.

SECTION TWO: Functions of the Liver

5. Examine Table 23-1. Major functions of the liver. If Rachel were to develop congestive heart failure, how would the liver respond?
   It would distend to take in the increased circulating blood volume.

   What liver related assessments, made by the nurse, would support presence of CHF?
   RUQ tenderness; Liver may be palpable

5. If Rachel had iron deficiency anemia, what role could her dysfunctional liver have played in this problem?
   The liver stores iron, as ferritin. When the liver is damaged, it can result in decreased levels of serum iron, thus contributing to iron deficiency anemia.

6. Rachel's liver dysfunction has significantly reduced the number of Kupffer's cells. What impact can this have on her outcomes?
   The Kupffer's cells are major macrophages that cleanse the blood volume of bacteria. Inability to properly cleanse the blood could allow contaminated blood to remain in the circulation, which could precipitate septicemia and/or peritonitis.

SECTION THREE: Evaluation of Liver Function Through Laboratory Tests

---

Rachel has liver enzyme and isoenzyme levels drawn.

---

7. How do enzyme levels reflect liver function?
   Enzymes are catalysts that help carry out cellular functions. Intracellular enzymes are generally found in several types of cells. When tissue are damaged, the enzymes escape from the damaged

cells and some moved into the circulation. By measuring the enzymes that are usually found in liver cells, one can indirectly measure damage to tissue.

8. What diagnostic advantages do isoenzymes have over their parent enzymes? Give examples of isoenzymes involved in liver functions.

They are more specific to a particular cell type. Certain ALT isoenzymes and LDH isoenzymes exist predominately in liver tissue. Examples: ALT isoenzymes – 5'-N, GGT, and OCT. LDH isoenzymes 4 and 5. Elevated levels of these isoenzymes are more diagnostic of a liver problem.

> **Rachel has additional laboratory testing done, with the following results: Total bilirubin = 27.3 mg/dL; Serum Albumin = 2.2 g/dL; PT = 14.8 seconds; Ammonia - 42 µg/dL.**

9. Why do bilirubin levels increase?

Normally, the liver converts unconjugated bilirubin into conjugated bilirubin (a water soluble form) that can be excreted through the feces. Dysfunction of the liver can decrease the liver's ability to convert bilirubin to its excretable form, thus it continues to circulate and levels continue to rise.

10. Rachel's ammonia level is high normal at this point. Where does the ammonia come from?

From deamination (breakdown) of amino-acids during protein catabolism.

11. Rachel's serum albumin is low. Consider what you know about the multisystem implications of low albumin. What clinical findings will you monitor her for and why?

Low serum albumin causes fluid shifts due to low osmotic pressure. Fluid leaves the intravascular compartment and third spaces, causing generalized edema. Severely low albumin can cause pulmonary edema.

SECTION FOUR: Acute Hepatitis

12. <u>True</u> / ***False*** (circle one). Acute hepatitis is most commonly caused by a bacterial infection.

> **Rachel is diagnosed with acute hepatitis secondary to acetaminophen toxicity**

13. In the space provided, match the description, to the correct type of hepatitis. Some will have several correct responses.

TYPE		DESCRIPTION
_B,F_ Hepatitis A		A. not a complete virus; requires surface antigen of hepatitis
_D,E,G_ Hepatitis B		B. transmission is via fecal-oral route
_C,D_ Hepatitis C		C. associated with increased risk for chronic liver disease
_A___ Hepatitis D		D. transmission is via blood serum or body fluids
_B___ Hepatitis E		E. at-risk group is similar to that of H.I.V.
		F. transmission is via contaminated food or water
		G. transmission is via contaminated needles or body fluids

14. Rachel's category of acute hepatitis is "submassive hepatic necrosis". How does this category differ from "classic hepatitis"?

It is more severe and more generalized, with wider necrotic activity. Some hepatic tissue collapses, losing its functional integrity. Tissue fibrosis may develop.

15. If she develops cholestatis hepatitis, what clinical findings will develop? *Jaundice, dark urine, clay colored stools, serum bilirubin of > 20-30 mg/dL.*

SECTION FIVE: Acute Hepatic Failure

> **Rachel's condition worsens. She is tentatively diagnosed with acute liver failure.**

16. Rachel's liver failure has most likely resulted from what? *hepatotoxins (acetaminophen)*

17. Rachel develops hepatic encephalopathy. It is currently being staged. Her current status is as follows: she is lethargic and drowsy. She has slurred speech and she is disoriented. This clinical presentation would place her at what stage of hepatic encephalopathy? *Stage II*

18. As Rachel's carbohydrate metabolism becomes impaired, the nurse can expect increasing hyperglycemia / *hypoglycemia* (circle one).

SECTION SIX: Complications of Hepatic Dysfunction

19. While she is in liver failure, Rachel is at risk for developing certain complications. In the table below, fill in the major associated clinical findings related to each of the common complications of liver dysfunction.

Complication	Major Associated Clinical Findings
Hepatic encephalopathy	*Decreased neurologic function*
Portal hypertension	*In acute hepatic failure: congested splanchnic organs* *In chronic hepatic dysfunction: develop esophageal varices*
Esophageal varices	*Seen in chronic hepatic dysfunction; varices are prone to rupture, causing hemorrhage*
Ascites	*A clinical finding*
Hepatorenal syndrome	*Findings associated with acute renal failure in presence of liver failure*
Infection	*Development of clinical manifestations of sepsis, peritonitis*

SECTION SEVEN: Medical Management

20. True / *False* (circle one). The medical treatment for viral hepatitis is composed of a specific drug regimen.

21. Briefly describe interventions that reduce ammonia toxins.
    Protein intake is significantly reduced or eliminated. In particular, aromatic amino acids need to be eliminated while branched-chain amino acid intake may continue to be taken in. Neomycin (PO) may be ordered to reduce ammonia-producing intestinal bacteria. Lactulose is often ordered to reduce absorption of ammonia from the bowel; it is also used for its laxative effect. Rapid stool elimination increases ammonia removal from the bowel.

22. To help protect Rachel from developing GI bleeding, the nurse can anticipate what type of therapy?
    Histamine antagonists or antacids; coagulopathy is controlled through vitamin K (and possible blood products)

23. Although in Rachel's situation bleeding esophageal varices are not likely, if it was believed that she was at risk for developing them, what general preventive therapy could the nurse anticipate?
    Control of her portal pressure is crucial. This may be done with Nitroglycerin, Vasopressin, or Terlipressin. If necessary, sclerotherapy might be performed, or shunt surgery.

SECTION EIGHT: Nursing Implications

24. A major focus of the nursing assessment of the patient with hepatic dysfunction is monitoring for signs and symptoms of ___*multisystem complications*_____.

25. During Rachel's latest assessment, the nurse observed involuntary tremors in Rachel's hands. What is the called, and what complication is it associated with?
     Asterixis (liver flap); Stage II hepatic encephalopathy

26. Rachel's skin has become extremely dry and flaky and her skin turgor is poor. These integumentary assessments are caused by:
     elevated levels of circulating hepatotoxins and fluid shifts

27. Rachel's breathing pattern is abnormally shallow and rapid. What pathophysiologic events may account for this altered breathing pattern?
     The presence of ascites can increase pressure on the diaphragm; general weakness; pleural effusion; and impaired thought processes all can contribute to breathing alterations.

28. Rachel is at increased risk for infection. Why is this a potential problem?
     As protein levels decrease, she can develop leukopenia. In addition, splenic hyperactivity can destroy blood cells.

Take Home Case
Module 24: Altered Glucose Metabolism

STUDENT NAME: _____. Date: _____

DIRECTIONS:

In narrative form, complete the following questions or statements based on the Module reading assignment. To better comprehend this material, it is best to answer the items in your own words rather than copying answers from the text. By doing so, you can evaluate what you actually understand.

Required Reading: *High Acuity Nursing, 2nd ed.* -- Module 24: Altered Glucose Metabolism
****

SITUATION: R. U. Quick is an insulin dependent diabetic. He was diagnosed with this condition as a child. Mr. Quick self-administers 24 units of Regular and 24 units of NPH insulin SQ every morning

SECTION ONE: Normal Glucose Metabolism

1. Briefly explain the difference between insulin-dependent cells and noninsulin-dependent cells. What is the major organ that is noninsulin-dependent?

2. Where is insulin produced?

3. Why is glucagon called the "hyperglycemic factor"? Where is it secreted from?

4. When serum glucose is low, the _____ nervous system is stimulated, which in turn, stimulates the adrenals to secrete the hormone _____.

5. Describe how insulin lowers circulating blood glucose levels by moving glucose into cells.

SECTION TWO: The Effects of Insulin on Metabolism

6. When Mr. Quick takes his insulin, it has what effect on his metabolism? Complete the table as directed:

Type of Metabolism	Effects of Insulin
Glucose	
Fat	
Protein	

7. <u>True / False</u> (circle one) During Mr. Quick's normal activities, muscle tissue use fatty acids for the major source of energy.

8. The organ primarily responsible for glucose storage is the _____.

SECTION THREE: The Effects of Insulin Deficit

9. If Mr. Quick develops an insulin deficit, his body will break down fat, a process called _____, to meet his energy needs. When fats are used for energy, they are used in the form of

   _____.

10. Which type of nutrient, when used as the primary energy source, ultimately converts into ketone bodies?

11. Mr. Quick's insulin deficit causes serum glucose levels to _____ which _____ plasma osmotic pressure. This causes body fluids to shift from _____ into the _____ compartment, which eventually causes _____ dehydration.

SECTION FOUR: Types of Diabetes Mellitus

4. Compare the terms absolute insulin deficit and relative insulin deficit. Which type of deficit would Mr. Quick most likely have?

5. Which type of diabetes is less apt to develop elevated ketones during times of insulin deficit?

SECTION FIVE: Hypoglycemic Coma

Mr. Quick develops hypoglycemia.

6. Although hypoglycemia is often clinically defined on the basis of the serum glucose, what do we know about the symptoms of hypoglycemia?

7. Mr. Quick's hypoglycemic clinical presentation has two major underlying effects, in the space provided, state the reasons for these effects.

Underlying Effects	*Reason for Effect*
• Central Nervous System	
• Catecholamine	

8. If Mr. Quick developed his hypoglycemia slowly, the nurse can anticipate seeing predominately which types of symptoms? Give examples of associated symptoms.

9. How does treatment change based on whether or not Mr. Quick remains conscious throughout his hypoglycemic episode?

SECTION SIX: Diabetic Ketoacidosis

> **Mr. Quick has been hospitalized for a large right lower extremity cellulitis and diabetic ketoacidosis (DKA).**

10. Mr. Quick's acute infection placed him at risk for which acid-base disturbance?

11. Explain the pathophysiologic events causing his acid-base disturbance, including the accompanying clinical findings you would expect to see.

12. There are three underlying problems that are the basis for the clinical presentation of the DKA patient. In the table provided, cluster the appropriate clinical findings with their corresponding underlying problem:

Underlying Problem	*Associated Clinical Findings*
• Hyperglycemia	
• Metabolic Acidosis	
• Osmotic Diuresis	

13. Mr. Quick is becoming severely dehydrated. Briefly explain the chain of events surrounding this DKA related problem.

14. Mr. Quick's serum electrolytes are as follows: $Na^+ = 128$, $K^+ = 2.8$, $Cl^- = 90$, and $HCO_3^- = 14$. What type of anion gap does he have (high or normal)?

15. Briefly explain how measuring anion gap is clinically helpful in diagnosing DKA?

16. What is the most common precipitating factor for development of DKA.

17. List the medical treatment plan for DKA:

18. Briefly explain why it is crucial to correct the underlying cause of the DKA.

19. List four common nursing diagnoses commonly associated with diabetic ketoacidosis:

SECTION SEVEN: Hyperglycemic Hyperosmolar Nonketotic Coma

20. As a type I diabetic, is Mr. Quick a likely candidate for HHNC? Why or why not?

21. Briefly describe the difference between DKA and Hyperosmolar hyperosmotic nonketotic coma (HHNC):

22. What is DKA-Hyperosmolar Syndrome? When should it be suspected?

SECTION EIGHT: Exogenous Insulin Therapy

23. Why has exogenous insulin usage rapidly moved toward use of synthetic insulins?

24. What general factors will increase Mr. Quick's insulin dosage requirements?

Mr. Quick required 8 units or Regular insulin SQ to treat a finger stick glucose of 305 mg/dL at 11 AM.

---

25. When would you expect peak effects of his insulin?

26. Mr Quick also receives NPH insulin at 8:00 AM every morning. During what time frame will the nurse need to monitor him the closest for the clinical manifestations of hypoglycemia due to his NPH?

27. While Mr. Quick's cellulitis remains active, he is placed on sliding scale insulin coverage. This term refers to:

SECTION NINE: Acute Care Implications of Chronic Complications

28. What are the acute care implications of the following chronic complications associated with diabetes?

Chronic Complication	Acute Care Implications
Peripheral neuropathies	
Retinopathy	
Nephropathy	
Peripheral vascular disease	
Increase risk of Infection	

Take Home Case
Module 24: Altered Glucose Metabolism
Instructor Guide

DIRECTIONS:
In narrative form, complete the following questions or statements based on the Module reading assignment. To better comprehend this material, it is best to answer the items in your own words rather than copying answers from the text. By doing so, you can evaluate what you actually understand.

Required Reading: *High Acuity Nursing, 2nd ed.* -- Module 24: Altered Glucose Metabolism
****

SITUATION: R. U. Quick is an insulin dependent diabetic. He was diagnosed with this condition as a child. Mr. Quick self-administers 24 units of Regular and 24 units of NPH insulin SQ every morning

SECTION ONE: Normal Glucose Metabolism
1. Briefly explain the difference between insulin-dependent cells and noninsulin-dependent cells. What is the major organ that is noninsulin-dependent?
    Insulin dependent cells require insulin to transport glucose into the cells while noninsulin dependent cells, such as exists in the brain, can take glucose across the cell membrane into the cell directly.

2. Where is insulin produced? *Beta cells of islets of Langerhans in pancreas*

3. Why is glucagon called the "hyperglycemic factor"? Where is it secreted from?
    Because it the major hormone responsible for raising serum glucose levels. It is secreted from alpha cells of the islets of Langerhans in the pancreas.

4. When serum glucose is low, the __*sympathetic*___ nervous system is stimulated, which in turn, stimulates the adrenals to secrete the hormone _*epinephrine*__.

5. Describe how insulin lowers circulating blood glucose levels by moving glucose into cells.
    Insulin binds to a carrier protein on the cell membrane. The carrier protein, with insulin, facilitates glucose diffusion across the cell membrane

SECTION TWO: The Effects of Insulin on Metabolism
6. When Mr. Quick takes his insulin, it has what effect on his metabolism? Complete the table as directed:

Type of Metabolism	Effects of Insulin
Glucose	• *facilitates cellular uptake of glucose* • *assists in conversion of glucose to glycogen for storage in liver*
Fat	• *facilitates use of glucose, thus sparing fat* • *promotes synthesis of fatty acids* • *inhibits fatty acid release* • *facilitates glucose transport into fat cells for fatty acid synthesis*
Protein	• *facilitates transport of amino acids across cell membranes* • *promotes protein synthesis* • *decreases protein catabolism*

7. *True* / False (circle one) During Mr. Quick's normal activities, muscle tissue use fatty acids for the major source of energy.
8. The organ primarily responsible for glucose storage is the ___*liver*__.

SECTION THREE: The Effects of Insulin Deficit

9. If Mr. Quick develops an insulin deficit, his body will break down fat, a process called __*lipolysis*__, to meet his energy needs. When fats are used for energy, they are used in the form of __*free fatty acids*_.

10. Which type of nutrient, when used as the primary energy source, ultimately converts into ketone bodies? *fats*

11. Mr. Quick's insulin deficit causes serum glucose levels to __*increase*___ which __*increases*___ plasma osmotic pressure. This causes body fluids to shift from __*tissue*__ into the __*intravascular*__ compartment, which eventually causes __*intracellular*__ dehydration.

SECTION FOUR: Types of Diabetes Mellitus

12. Compare the terms absolute insulin deficit and relative insulin deficit. Which type of deficit would Mr. Quick most likely have?

    An absolute insulin deficit means that the beta cells produce no insulin. This type of diabetes is associated with type I (insulin-dependent) diabetes. Relative insulin deficit means that the beta cells still produce some amount of insulin but in less than normal quantities. This type of deficit is associated with type II (non-insulin-dependent) diabetes. Mr. Quick most likely has an absolute insulin deficit.

13. Which type of diabetes is less apt to develop elevated ketones during times of insulin deficit? *Type I*

SECTION FIVE: Hypoglycemic Coma

Mr. Quick develops hypoglycemia.

14. Although hypoglycemia is often clinically defined on the basis of the serum glucose, what do we know about the symptoms of hypoglycemia?

    The symptoms can develop a higher serum glucose levels, particularly when the glucose drops rapidly.

15. Mr. Quick's hypoglycemic clinical presentation has two major underlying effects, in the space provided, state the reasons for these effects.

Underlying Effects	Reason for Effect
• Central Nervous System	◆ *The CNS is a non-insulin-dependent system. It requires glucose for energy, to carry on normal functioning. When there is a glucose deficit, CNS function rapidly becomes impaired.*
• Catecholamine	◆ *Lack of glucose in the circulation triggers the stress hormones. Catecholamines are released to stimulate release of alternate glucose sources.*

16. If Mr. Quick developed his hypoglycemia slowly, the nurse can anticipate seeing predominately which types of symptoms? Give examples of associated symptoms.

    Central Nervous System manifestations will predominate. For example: Increasing changes in mentation; altered speech and balance; decreasing level of consciousness.

17. How does treatment change based on whether or not Mr. Quick remains conscious throughout his hypoglycemic episode?

    If he remains conscious, he should be given appropriate food and/or fluids orally since sugars are rapidly absorbed through the GI tract. If he is unconscious, he will require parenteral administration of glucose.

SECTION SIX: Diabetic Ketoacidosis

> **Mr. Quick has been hospitalized for a large right lower extremity cellulitis and diabetic ketoacidosis (DKA).**

18. Mr. Quick's acute infection placed him at risk for which acid-base disturbance? *Metabolic acidosis*

19. Explain the pathophysiologic events causing his acid-base disturbance, including the accompanying clinical findings you would expect to see.

> *The stress of the infection causes an increase in serum glucose but the glucose cannot be transferred into the cells. To supply a source of energy, the body turns to free fatty acids as its primary energy source. Free fatty acids are broken down faster than they can be converted into glucose, forming ketone bodies (acetoacetic acid, β-hydroxybutric acid, and acetone). Ketone bodies decrease the pH, leading to metabolic acidosis.*

20. There are three underlying problems that are the basis for the clinical presentation of the DKA patient. In the table provided, cluster the appropriate clinical findings with their corresponding underlying problem:

Underlying Problem	*Associated Clinical Findings*
• Hyperglycemia	Elevated serum and urine glucose
• Metabolic Acidosis	Decreased serum pH; Elevated ketones (serum & urine); Acidotic HCO_3; ketone (fruity) breath; Kussmaul breathing
• Osmotic Diuresis	Polyuria; polydipsia; dehydration; hypotension; electrolyte abnormalities; increased serum osmolarity

21. Mr. Quick is becoming severely dehydrated. Briefly explain the chain of events surrounding this DKA related problem.

> *Since fluid is pulled from an area of low concentration to an area of higher concentration across a semi-permeable membrane, elevated serum glucose attracts extravascular fluids into the intravascular compartment to dilute the higher glucose concentration. As glucose and fluid levels increase, the kidneys increase their excretion to rid the body of the excesses. This leads to loss of fluid and electrolytes.*

22. Mr. Quick's serum electrolytes are as follows: $Na^+ = 128$, $K^+ = 2.8$, $Cl^- = 90$, and $HCO_3^- = 14$. What type of anion gap does he have (high or normal)? *High*

23. Briefly explain how measuring anion gap is clinically helpful in diagnosing DKA.

> *It helps differentiate etiologies of acidotic states. In particular, it helps to isolate DKA from other types of acidosis. DKA is a high anion gap (> 17 mEq/L) acidosis, as are starvation and lactic acidosis.*

24. What is the most common precipitating factor for development of DKA? *acute infection*

25. List the medical treatment plan for DKA:

> *IV therapy; insulin therapy; sodium bicarbonate therapy; electrolyte replacement; correction of underlying problems' serial laboratory tests.*

26. Briefly explain why it is crucial to correct the underlying cause of the DKA?

> *Until the underlying stressor has been corrected, Mr. Quick will continue to produce increased quantities of glucose, maintaining a high demand metabolic state. This is why the insulin-dependent diabetic high acuity patient requires higher doses of exogenous insulin during illness and the non-insulin-dependent patient often requires temporary insulin supplementation.*

27. List four common nursing diagnoses commonly associated with diabetic ketoacidosis:
    1) fluid volume deficit 2) altered nutrition: less than body requirements; 3) PC: electrolyte imbalances; 4) PC: metabolic acidosis

SECTION SEVEN: Hyperglycemic Hyperosmolar Nonketotic Coma
28. As a type I diabetic, is Mr. Quick a likely candidate for HHNC? Why or why not?
    No, he is more likely to develop DKA. HHNC is most commonly seen in the type II diabetic because it is associated with a relative insulin deficit rather than an absolute deficit. The type II diabetic can produce sufficient insulin to prevent (or minimize) ketone build-up but insufficient insulin to handle the increased levels of glucose during a period of stress.

29. Briefly describe the difference between DKA and Hyperosmolar hyperosmotic nonketotic coma (HHNC):
    The differences are mostly related to the degree of severity: DKA = rapid onset while HHNC = slower onset. Lack of significant ketones (and lack of ketone breath) and normal anion gap in HHNC are major differences. Hyperglycemia and hyperosmolarity, and osmotic diuresis are all more severe in HHNC. The neurologic signs noted in HHNC are more severe (deep coma and seizures). HHNC is associated with a much higher mortality rate than DKA because of it devastatingly severe effects.

30. What is DKA-Hyperosmolar Syndrome? When should it be suspected?
    A syndrome of signs and symptoms that exhibit aspects of both DKA and HHNC. It should be suspected when a patient is admitted with DKA but is in a comatose state.

SECTION EIGHT: Exogenous Insulin Therapy
31. Why has exogenous insulin usage rapidly moved toward use of synthetic insulins?
    Because the synthetic insulins are structured essentially identical to human insulin thus making them well accepted by the body. This cannot be said for earlier animal based insulins.

32. What general factors will increase Mr. Quick's insulin dosage requirements?
    His infection; exercise; acute illness; nutritional support; steroid therapy

> **Mr. Quick required 8 units or Regular insulin SQ to treat a finger stick glucose of 305 mg/dL at 11 AM.**

33. When would you expect peak effects of his insulin?
    Between 1:00 PM and 3:00 PM (since the peak effect for regular insulin is 2 to 4 hours).

34. Mr. Quick also receives NPH insulin at 8:00 AM every morning. During what time frame will the nurse need to monitor him the closest for the clinical manifestations of hypoglycemia due to his NPH?
    Between 2 PM and 8 PM that afternoon

35. While Mr. Quick's cellulitis remains active, he is placed on sliding scale insulin coverage. This term refers to:
    A prescribed regimen of scaled regular insulin dosing based on blood glucose levels which are drawn at regular intervals.

SECTION NINE: Acute Care Implications of Chronic Complications
36. What are the acute care implications of the following chronic complications associated with diabetes?

Chronic Complication	Acute Care Implications
Peripheral neuropathies	• *Assess for presence – may mask symptoms.* • *Protect from tissue injury, including hyperthermic*
Retinopathy	• *Assess for presence of visual impairment.* • *Alter environment and interactions based on level of impairment, if present.*

Chronic Complication	Acute Care Implications
Nephropathy	• *Monitor renal function closely.* • *Be aware of drug therapy that is nephrotoxic*
Peripheral vascular disease	• *Assess skin integrity closely* • *Careful limb positioning* • *Excellent skin hygiene*
Increase risk of Infection	• *Assess for presence of infection* • *Aggressively treat infection* • *Assess wounds for healing status* • *Maintain good control of serum glucose levels*

Take Home Case
Module 26: Acute Renal Dysfunction

DIRECTIONS:

In narrative form, complete the following questions or statements based on the Module reading assignment. To better comprehend this material, it is best to answer the items in your own words rather than copying answers from the text. By doing so, you can evaluate what you actually understand.

Required Reading: *High Acuity Nursing, 2ⁿᵈ ed.* -- Module 26: Acute Renal Dysfunction

****

> **SITUATION:** Andrew B. is a 63 year old retired assembly line worker with a past medical history of two previous myocardial infarctions, and congestive heart failure. He is now complaining of frequent chest pains, dyspnea on exertion, and swelling of his lower extremities. His blood pressure on admission is 74/46. The nurse notes that Andrew's urine output has only been 45 mL for the past two hours.

SECTION ONE: Normal Kidney Function

1. The functional unit of the kidney is the _____. It is composed of three structures, the

    _____, _____, and _____.

2. In order for glomerular filtration to occur, what two factors must be present?

3. Andrew is hypotensive. Briefly explain how this cardiovascular problem can affect his kidney function.

SECTION TWO: Influences of Body Systems on Renal Function

3. Assuming Andrew's nervous and endocrine systems are intact, what mechanisms to they use to attempt to maintain renal perfusion in the face of hemodynamic compromise?

4. Briefly explain in what way autoregulation is important to renal blood flow

SECTION THREE: Causes of Acute Renal Failure

.3. According to Andrew's recent history, which type of acute renal failure is he initially at most risk of developing and why?

> On admission, Andrew's BUN was 15 and his creatinine was 1.2.
> On day #3, Andrew's lab values were as follows:

> BUN = 58, Creatinine = 5.4, Na = 130, K = 6.6, Cl = 90, CO_2 = 18, Ca = 3.0, Mg = 1.8, and PO_4 = 6.5
> Andrew's urinary output decreased to < 15 mL per hour and he experienced fluid overload. Lasix did to improve his urinary output. His hypotension was managed with a Dopamine and he was treated with Gentamicin for a bacteremia.

4. Considering these latest changes, what specifically has Andrew most likely developed?

5. Briefly explain Andrew's risk factors which have contributed to the development of his renal dysfunction:

6. Andrew's pattern of renal lab findings are consistent with and initial _____ failure secondary to hypoperfusion which became a(n) _____ failure.

SECTION FOUR: The Stages of Acute Renal Failure

6. It is now two days following Andrew's hypotensive episode. His urinary output has been less than 15 mL per hour for the last eight hours. Based on this information, what stage of acute renal failure is he in?

7. What criteria can be used to help determined when Andrew goes into the early diuretic stage of his renal failure?

8. When Andrew is discharged from the hospital, in the convalescent stage of his renal failure, what drug related precaution should the nurse instruct him about?

SECTION FIVE: Assessment of Acute Renal Dysfunction

9. Andrew is at risk for developing multiple system clinical manifestations due to his acute renal failure. What clinical manifestations would you expect to see based on these multisystem effects, and what is the underlying cause of these findings?

Effects	Causes	Clinical Manifestations
Neurologic		•
Cardiovascular		•
Pulmonary		

Effects	Causes	Clinical Manifestations
Gastrointestinal		
Hematopoietic		
Integumentary		
Skeletal		

10. BUN and creatinine are the two most common laboratory tests used to determine renal function. Of the two, which is more reflective of renal function. Why?

11. Since Andrew is in acute renal failure, as his serum urea nitrogen and creatinine increase, you would expect his urine urea nitrogen and creatinine to _____.

12. His serum albumin levels are dropping. Why do you think this is occurring?

SECTION SIX: The Effect of Acute Renal Failure on Fluid and Electrolyte Balance

13. During the oliguric/anuric stage of his ARF, you would expect Andrew to be experiencing the clinical manifestations consistent with <u>fluid volume excess / fluid volume deficit</u> (circle one).

14. During the oliguric/anuric stage of his ARF, Andrew has serum electrolytes drawn. Overall, you would anticipate that his electrolytes will <u>increase / decrease</u> (circle one) with the exception of _____ and _____.

15. Andrew is at high risk for developing metabolic acidosis. What factors contribute to this problem in the presence of renal failure?

SECTION SEVEN: Management of the Patient in Acute Renal Failure

16. Andrew's medical management will largely focus on four major potential complications associated with his renal dysfunction. Complete the following table. It will help to summarize major points regarding management of A.R.F.

Complication	Treatment	Common Related Nursing Diagnoses
Catabolic Processes		
Electrolyte / Acid-base Imbalance		
Infection		

SECTION EIGHT: Dialysis, an Acute Renal Failure Treatment Modality

17. When it was first suspected that Andrew might be going into early stages of acute renal failure, what diagnostic interventions might be performed to help differentiate a prerenal problem from an intrarenal problem?

It is determined that Andrew has an intrarenal type of renal failure. It has now been four days since the onset of his failure and his fluid and electrolyte imbalances require that dialysis be initiated.

18. Briefly explain the process on which dialysis is based:

19. True / False (circle one). Dialysis is used to correct the underlying renal dysfunction.

Since Andrew's condition is fairly stable, it is decided to use hemodialysis.

20. What are the most common temporary venous access sites?

21. Briefly explain how Andrew's blood is cleansed during hemodialysis:

22. True / False (circle one). Dialysate solutions can draw fluid and solutes from, as well as give solutes to the patient.

Take Home Case
Module 26: Acute Renal Dysfunction
Instructor Guide

DIRECTIONS:

In narrative form, complete the following questions or statements based on the Module reading assignment. To better comprehend this material, it is best to answer the items in your own words rather than copying answers from the text. By doing so, you can evaluate what you actually understand.

Required Reading: *High Acuity Nursing, 2nd ed.* -- Module 26: Acute Renal Dysfunction
****

> **SITUATION:** Andrew B. is a 63 year old retired assembly line worker with a past medical history of two previous myocardial infarctions, and congestive heart failure. He is now complaining of frequent chest pains, dyspnea on exertion, and swelling of his lower extremities. His blood pressure on admission is 74/46. The nurse notes that Andrew's urine output has only been 45 mL for the past two hours.

SECTION ONE: Normal Kidney Function

1. The functional unit of the kidney is the __*nephron*__. It is composed of three structures, the

   __*glomerulus*__, __*tubular apparatus*__, and __*collecting duct*__.

2. In order for glomerular filtration to occur, what two factors must be present?

   Adequate blood volume in the intravascular space and adequate hydrostatic pressure from cardiac output and vascular resistance

3. Andrew is hypotensive. Briefly explain how this cardiovascular problem can affect his kidney function?
   A hypotensive episode decreases cardiac output. If cardiac output drops too low, the kidneys will not receive adequate blood flow to perfuse the tissues, leading to tissue ischemia and damage.

SECTION TWO: Influences of Body Systems on Renal Function

3. Assuming Andrew's nervous and endocrine systems are intact, what mechanisms to they use to attempt to maintain renal perfusion in the face of hemodynamic compromise?
   The sympathetic nervous system has baroreceptors (sensitive to BP changes), chemoreceptors (sensitive to CO_2 and H^+ changes), and osmoreceptors (sensitive to water osmolality changes). In addition, fluid balance is partially regulated by the thirst mechanism. The endocrine system manipulates renal function through its two hormones: ADH and aldosterone.

4. Briefly explain in what way autoregulation is important to renal blood flow
   It regulates renal blood flow resistance to maintain a normal GFR and resistance of flow of blood under varying blood pressure conditions.

SECTION THREE: Causes of Acute Renal Failure

3. According to Andrew's recent history, which type of acute renal failure is he initially at most risk of developing and why? *prenal acute renal failure*

> On admission, Andrew's BUN was 15 and his creatinine was 1.2.
> On day #3, Andrew's lab values were as follows:
>   BUN = 58, Creatinine = 5.4, Na = 130, K = 6.6, Cl = 90, CO_2 = 18, Ca = 3.0,
>   Mg = 1.8, and PO_4 = 6.5

> **Andrew's urinary output decreased to < 15 mL per hour and he experienced fluid overload. Lasix did to improve his urinary output. His hypotension was managed with a Dopamine and he was treated with Gentamicin for a bacteremia.**

4. Considering these latest changes, what specifically has Andrew most likely developed?
    Acute Tubular Necrosis

5. Briefly explain Andrew's risk factors which have contributed to the development of his renal dysfunction:
    His hypotensive episode decreased his cardiac output and decreased renal perfusion. This, in turn, leads to renal tissue ischemia and acute tubular necrosis.

6. Andrew's pattern of renal lab findings are consistent with and initial __*prerenal*__ failure secondary to
    hypoperfusion which became a(n) _*intrarenal*_ failure.

SECTION FOUR: The Stages of Acute Renal Failure

6. It is now two days following Andrew's hypotensive episode. His urinary output has been less than 15 mL per hour for the last eight hours. Based on this information, what stage of acute renal failure is he in?
    Oliguric/Anuric

7. What criteria can be used to help determined when Andrew goes into the early diuretic stage of his renal failure?
    U/O increases to > 400 mL/24 hours; BUN and creatinine are still rising

8. When Andrew is discharged from the hospital, in the convalescent stage of his renal failure, what drug related precaution should the nurse instruct him about?
    It is crucial that he avoid nephrotoxic agents – He should inform any person prescribing medications about his ARF episode. He should also consult with appropriate health professionals prior to taking OTC agents.

SECTION FIVE: Assessment of Acute Renal Dysfunction

9. Andrew is at risk for developing multiple system clinical manifestations due to his acute renal failure. What clinical manifestations would you expect to see based on these multisystem effects, and what is the underlying cause of these findings?

Effects	*Causes*	*Clinical Manifestations*
Neurologic	*Accumulation of nitrogenous waste products*	• *decreasing responsiveness* • *seizures* • *itching, tingling, numbness, twitching of extremities*
Cardiovascular	*Fluid volume excess; increased renin production; electrolyte imbalances; H^+ excess*	• *hypertension* • *cardiac arrhythmias* • *peripheral edema* • *C.H.F. clinical findings*
Pulmonary	*Decreased responsiveness; weakness; thick secretions; decreased cough; decreased pulm. macrophage activity*	• *adventitious breath sounds* • *pneumonia*
Gastrointestinal	*Electrolyte imbalances & increasing levels of uremic toxins*	• *weight loss* • *positive guaiac stools* • *anorexia, nausea / vomiting* • *constipation or diarrhea*

Effects	Causes	Clinical Manifestations
Hematopoietic	*Reduced production of erythropoietin; impaired platelet function*	• *anemia* • *fatigue, weakness* • *pale mucous membranes*
Integumentary	*Uremic toxins excreted via skin; dysfunctional platelets*	• *pruritus* • *thin hair & brittle, thin nails* • *pale, dry, dull, yellow skin* • *bruising*
Skeletal	*Decreased absorption of Calcium due to inability of kidneys to metabolize vit. D.*	• *long term skeletal disorders*

10. BUN and creatinine are the two most common laboratory tests used to determine renal function. Of the two, which is more reflective of renal function. Why?

> *Creatinine; BUN is the end product of protein metabolism while creatinine is the end product of muscle metabolism. Of these two, muscle metabolism is more stable since less factors alter it. Therefore, since BUN reflects the less reliable type of metabolism, it is considered less reliable It is less specific to kidney function.*

11. Since Andrew is in acute renal failure, as his serum urea nitrogen and creatinine increase, you would expect his urine urea nitrogen and creatinine to ___*decrease*___.

12. His serum albumin levels are dropping. Why do you think this is occurring?

> *The damage renal tubules allow proteins to escape, thus decreasing plasma protein in the serum and increasing urine levels.*

SECTION SIX: The Effect of Acute Renal Failure on Fluid and Electrolyte Balance

13. During the oliguric/anuric stage of his ARF, you would expect Andrew to be experiencing the clinical manifestations consistent with *fluid volume excess* / fluid volume deficit (circle one).

14. During the oliguric/anuric stage of his ARF, Andrew has serum electrolytes drawn. Overall, you would anticipate that his electrolytes will *increase* / decrease (circle one) with the exception of __*calcium*_ and *phosphate*_.

15. Andrew is at high risk for developing metabolic acidosis. What factors contribute to this problem in the presence of renal failure?

> *Since the kidneys play a crucial part in maintaining acid-base balance through excretion of H^+, when kidney function is decreased, H^+ is not adequately eliminated, thus building up in the body. Compounding this problem is the loss or decrease of HCO_3 buffering capabilities (again secondary to renal damage).*

SECTION SEVEN: Management of the Patient in Acute Renal Failure

16. Andrew's medical management will largely focus on four major potential complications associated with his renal dysfunction. The following table will help to summarize major points regarding management.

Complication	Treatment	Common Related Nursing Diagnoses
Catabolic Processes	1) *Nutritional support* 2) *Diet restricted in protein, Na, K, and fluids, high in carbohydrates and fats, & essential amino acids*	1) *Altered nutrition: Less than body requirements* 2) *PC: GI bleeding* 3) *Alt. though processes*

Complication	Treatment	Common Related Nursing Diagnoses
	3) *Dialysis*	4) *Diarrhea* 5) *Constipation*
Electrolyte / Acid-base Imbalance	1. *Cation exchange resins* 2. *Na, HCO₃, insulin, hypertonic glucose – to drive K⁺ back into cells* 3. *Dialysis*	1. *PC: Metabolic acidosis* 2. *Electrolyte imbalance* 3. *Fluid volume excess*
Infection	1. *Antibiotic therapy* 2. *Minimal use of invasive lines / tubes* 3. *Culturing suspicious secretions/ excretions*	*High risk for infection*

SECTION EIGHT: Dialysis, an Acute Renal Failure Treatment Modality

17. When it was first suspected that Andrew might be going into early stages of acute renal failure, what diagnostic interventions might be performed to help differentiate a prerenal problem from an intrarenal problem?

    A diuretic challenge may be given. If the kidneys are able to respond, it is a prerenal problem. If there is no response, it is most likely an intrarenal problem.

It is determined that Andrew has an intrarenal type of renal failure. It has now been four days since the onset of his failure and his fluid and electrolyte imbalances require that dialysis be initiated.

---

18. Briefly explain the process on which dialysis is based:

    Diffusion. Dissolved particles are transported across a semipermeable membrane from one fluid compartment to another. Diffusion occurs down the concentration gradient – blood has a higher solute concentration than dialysis does.

19. <u>True</u> / ***False*** (circle one). Dialysis is used to correct the underlying renal dysfunction.

Since Andrew's condition is fairly stable, it is decided to use hemodialysis.

---

20. What are the most common temporary venous access sites? *subclavian vein or femoral vein*

21. Briefly explain how Andrew's blood is cleansed during hemodialysis:

    The patient's blood passes through the venous access and into a dialyzer. As the blood flows through the dialyzer, excess fluid and solutes are removed across the semipermeable membrane, and the filtered blood is returned to the patient.

22. ***True*** / <u>False</u> (circle one). Dialysate solutions can draw fluid and solutes from, as well as give solutes to the patient.

Case Studies
Diabetic Crises

Case Study A: Mrs. Sugarbacker

Mrs. Sugarbacker, 56 years old, is a patient in your facility for a probable bleeding gastrointestinal ulcer. Her history indicates that she has had dark bloody stool for a 2 week period. She denies nausea and vomiting although she has experienced a decreased appetite for the past month. She reports a 10# weight loss over the last 3 months. She is scheduled for a Barium Swallow tomorrow. Her past medical history is significant for insulin-dependent diabetes mellitus (IDDM) and hypertension. At home she has been self-administering NPH insulin (20 units), and Regular insulin (10 units) every morning. Her hypertension is currently diet controlled.

On Day Two:

The Barium Swallow is scheduled for 11 a.m. today. She has been NPO since midnight. At 0730 you administer her usual insulin dose and complete your initial shift assessment. The transport aide takes Mrs. Sugarbacker to special procedures at 1045. She returns at 12 noon. As the stretcher passes you in the hall, you note that she is lethargic, diaphoretic, and pale. She does not respond to commands when you enter her room.

1.	What additional data would you like to obtain and why?

2.	Cluster the clues and give your assessment of what is wrong with Mrs. Sugarbacker. Write a nursing diagnosis.

3.	Based on your assessment and nursing diagnosis, what would be your priority actions?

4.	What factors contributed to this condition?

5.	What are the pathological processes that produced her symptoms?

6.	When does the Regular insulin administered to Mrs. S. peak?

7.	When does the NPH insulin administered to Mrs. S. peak?

8.	When you prepared the insulin injection, you withdrew the regular insulin from the vial first, then withdrew the NPH into the same syringe. Comment on this.

9. The vials on insulin were labeled Humulin - R and Humulin-N. Was the proper medication administered?

10. How would you revise Mrs. S's treatment plan in the future if she is scheduled for surgery?

Case Study B: Nancy Porter-Hall

Nancy Porter-Hall, 37 years old., was found by her daughter in a stuporous condition. She was responsive only to light shaking. The emergency squad was called and Nancy was taken to the emergency department.

Upon arrival at the emergency department, the nurse's initial assessment reveals that Nancy is hot and dry. Her lips are dry and cracked. She is lethargic, moaning in response to sternal rubbing. The nurse notes that her respirations are rapid and she has a fruity odor to her breath. It is also noted that she is wearing a diabetic alert necklace. The nurse focuses in on a rapid assessment and obtains the following data:

A fingerstick glucose level is at the upper limits of the glucometer. Vital signs: BP = 80/40, HR = 118, R = 42, T = 101.8.

The nurse obtains an IV access and STAT labs are drawn with the following results:

Glucose	=	704						
Serum Ketones	=	+						
pH	=	7.0	Na	=	124	Hgb	=	12
PCO_2	=	17	K	=	6.2	Hct	=	36
PO_2	=	90	Cl	=	92	WBC	=	24
SaO_2	=	94%	CO_2	=	6			
HCO_3	=	4						

1.   Cluster the clues and determine your assessment of Nancy.

2.   Which type of diabetes is most frequently the cause of this condition?

3.   The House Officer orders blood, urine and sputum cultures, why?

4.   Explain the pathogenesis of Nancy's presentation:

   a.   Glucose of 704:

   b.   + Serum Ketones:

   c.   Metabolic acidosis:

   d.   Respirations of 42/minute:

   e.   Fruity odor to breath:

   f.   BP 80/40, HR 118, dry lips:

5.   What are the 4 main treatment objectives for Nancy?

6.   How would Nancy's glucose of 704 be treated?

7.   The House Officer (HO) does not order $NaHCO_3$ for her serum pH of 7.0, would you remind him to?

8.   The HO orders "KCl 20 mEq X 2 doses over 1 hour each, to begin in 3 hours". But her admission K was 6.2. Would you question this order?

9.   What is the IVF you should hang for Nancy?

10.   Nancy's BP was 80/40 on admission. The admission orders contain an order for Dopamine 12 mcg/kg/minute. Would you question this order?

Case C: Beau Jones

Beau Jones, a frail appearing 78 year old nursing home patient, is transferred to your hospital with the following history:

He is a Type II diabetic who has been diet controlled for five years. Four days ago, he developed flu-like symptoms, becoming very nauseated and was unable to take food or fluids. His physician ordered a high carbohydrate tube feeding to be initiated to prevent malnutrition and dehydration. Two days ago, the nurses noted that Mr. Jones had developed a decreased level of consciousness which has been progressively worsening. On admission to the hospital, Beau does not respond to anything but deep pain stimulation. His vital signs are as follows:

BP = 88/48, P = 126, R = 32 and shallow, T = 102

1. What available cues are there that would suggest that Beau is experiencing a diabetic crisis?

2. Based on his clinical presentation AND history, what is probably his medical diangosis?

DKA: _____
HHNC: _____
Hypoglycemic Coma: _____

3. What labs would be helpful in confirming this diagnosis and what findings would be expected? (Compare how the results would differ, based on each diagnosis)

Laboratory Data	DKA	HHNC

4. What other signs and symptoms would you anticipate related to his probable diagnosis?

5. What would be your PRIORITY nursing diagnoses based on this diagnosis? What expected patient outcomes will you evaluate? What PRIORITY nursing interventions would be appropriate during his crisis state?

#1 Nursing Diagnosis:
EPOs:

Priority Nursing Intervention(s):

#2 Nursing Diagnosis:
EPOs:

Priority Nursing Intervention(s):

#3 Nursing Diagnosis:
EPOs:

Priority Nursing Interventions(s):

6.   What population is at particular risk for development of HHNC?

7.   What is the pathological basis for HHNC?

Case Study
Diabetic Crises
Instructor Guide

Case Study A: Mrs. Sugarbacker

Please Note: The following case studies can take the place of a regular class format. Each case study discusses major concepts dealing with one of the three major diabetic crises.

Mrs. Sugarbacker, 56 years old, is a patient in your facility for a probable bleeding gastrointestinal ulcer. Her history indicates that she has had dark bloody stool for a 2 week period. She denies nausea and vomiting although she has experienced a decreased appetite for the past month. She reports a 10# weight loss over the last 3 months. She is scheduled for a Barium Swallow tomorrow. Her past medical history is significant for insulin-dependent diabetes mellitus (IDDM) and hypertension. At home she has been self-administering NPH insulin (20 units), and Regular insulin (10 units) every morning. Her hypertension is currently diet controlled.

On Day Two:

The Barium Swallow is scheduled for 11 a.m. today. She has been NPO since midnight. At 0730 you administer her usual insulin dose and complete your initial shift assessment. The transport aide takes Mrs. Sugarbacker to special procedures at 1045. She returns at 12 noon. As the stretcher passes you in the hall, you note that she is lethargic, diaphoretic, and pale. She does not respond to commands when you enter her room.

1.   What additional data would you like to obtain and why?
   > *VS: 140/80, HR 130, R 14, T 99.8 - reason would check -- she is diaphoretic and pale. It is important to know if it is related to a low BP.*
   > *Glasgow Coma Scale: EMV = 14. Reason would check -- she is lethargic and does not follow commands*
   > *finger stick glucose is 40. Reason would check -- history of IDDM*

2.   Cluster the clues and give your assessment of what is wrong with Mrs. Sugarbacker. Write a nursing diagnosis.
   > *Increased pulse; decreased EMV; decreased glucose; diaphoretic & pale (SNS response)*
   > *Hx of IDDM; Glucose = 40 (hypoglycemia = < 50)*
   > *Nsg Dx: Could use either 1) alt. in nutrition: less than body requirements; or 2) pot. for injury*

3.   Based on your assessment and nursing diagnosis, what would be your priority actions?
   > *1)   Someone should call the house officer or the patient's physician*
   > *2)   Someone should get 1/2 cup of orange juice or 2 sugar packets to provide 10 - 15 gm of glucose. In 5 minutes, check for increasing mental status.*
   > *3)   If EMV is ≤ 8, check for IV access or obtain one and administer 50% dextrose.*

4.   What factors contributed to this condition?
   > *NPO status of approximately 12 hours without food while administering her "usual" insulin dosage. Hypoglycemia can be caused by: more insulin than is needed; insufficient food taken in; decreased food absorption (such as nausea and vomiting)*

5.   What are the pathological processes that produced her symptoms?
   > *Activation of sympathetic nervous system: associated with increased pulse, diaphoresis and paleness. Decreased glucose stimulates the SNS to release epinephrine to stimulate the liver to initiate gluconeogenesis.*
   > *Central Nervous System: Hypoglycemia becomes symptomatic when there is insufficient*

glucose available to meet the CNS needs. Brain cells are not insulin dependent and take in glucose directly.

6. When does the Regular insulin administered to Mrs. S. peak?

    Her insulin was administered at 0730. Regular insulin peaks approximately 4 hours later, therefore it should have peaked at approximately 1130.

7. When does the NPH insulin administered to Mrs. S. peak?

    Her NPH was administered at 0730. NPH insulin peaks approximately 8 hours later, therefore it should have peaked at approximately 1530. NPH begins to take effect in 3-4 hours.

8. When you prepared the insulin injection, you withdrew the regular insulin from the vial first, then withdrew the NPH into the same syringe. Comment on this.

    The rule is clear then cloudy. Alphabetically clear comes before cloudy.

9. The vials on insulin were labeled Humulin - R and Humulin-N. Was the proper medication administered?

    There is no specification of the exact insulin order. It is important to know what type of insulin she is taking since they cannot be interchanged. This should have been clarified prior to administering.

10. How would you revise Mrs. S's treatment plan in the future if she is scheduled for surgery?

    1. An IDDM diabetic who is NPO and still receives insulin, needs glucose via some route (perhaps IV in her case)
    2. Her test could possibly have been scheduled early in the day to avoid prolonged NPO
    3. Her insulin order could have been adjusted via the physician -- especially her regular insulin dose. The nurse could have contacted the physician to clarify the situation. The regular insulin dose was the major problem in Mrs. S's case

Case Study B: Nancy Porter-Hall

Nancy Porter-Hall, 37 years old., was found by her daughter in a stuporous condition. She was responsive only to light shaking. The emergency squad was called and Nancy was taken to the emergency department.

Upon arrival at the emergency department, the nurse's initial assessment reveals that Nancy is hot and dry. Her lips are dry and cracked. She is lethargic, moaning in response to sternal rubbing. The nurse notes that her respirations are rapid and she has a fruity odor to her breath. It is also noted that she is wearing a diabetic alert necklace. The nurse focuses in on a rapid assessment and obtains the following data:

A fingerstick glucose level is at the upper limits of the glucometer. Vital signs: BP = 80/40, HR = 118, R = 42, T = 101.8.

The nurse obtains an IV access and STAT labs are drawn with the following results:

Glucose	=	704						
Serum Ketones	=	+						
pH	=	7.0	Na	=	124	Hgb	=	12
PCO_2	=	17	K	=	6.2	Hct	=	36
PO_2	=	90	Cl	=	92	WBC	=	24
SaO_2	=	94%	CO_2	=	6			
HCO_3	=	4						

1.   Cluster the clues and determine your assessment of Nancy.
Metabolic acidosis, increased respirations, fruity odor, glucose 704, positive ketones, dry and cracked lips (dehydrated), diabetic alert bracelet, reduced EMV.

2.   Which type of diabetes is most frequently the cause of this condition?
Her clinical presentation is consistent with DKA rather than HHNC. At 37 years of age, she is more likely a IDDM person. Her fruity breath, + ketones, metabolic acidosis all help distinguish DKA from HHNC.

3.   The House Officer orders blood, urine and sputum cultures, why?
Results: WBC = 24,000, T = 101.8. Other than omission of insulin, the No. 1 cause of DKA is infection.

4.   Explain the pathogenesis of Nancy's presentation:

a.   Glucose of 704: *Without insulin, there is no "bridge" to assist glucose into the cells, thereby allowing it to increase in the serum while the cells become glucose starved.*

b.   + Serum Ketones: *Inability of the cells to use glucose results in breakdown of fats. When fats are used as an energy source, ketones are released.*

c.   Metabolic acidosis: *ketones are a byproduct of fat metabolism and represent acid. As they increase in the serum, pH will drop.*

d.   Respirations of 42/minute: *As pH drops, the respiratory center is stimulated to increase the respiratory rate to help blow off CO_2. Kussmaul's breathing.*

e.   Fruity odor to breath: *Acetone is formed as part of the breakdown of fatty acids. Acetone is blown off with increased respiratory rate.*

f.   BP 80/40, HR 118, dry lips: *As glucose and ketones are excreted in the urine, they "pull" water with them. This is called osmotic diuresis. Diuresis may be severe, causing dehydration. The above data suggests dehydration.*

5.   What are the 4 main treatment objectives for Nancy?
       1.   Reduce serum glucose level
       2.   Replace electrolytes
       3.   Replace fluids
       4.   Treat the underlying cause (such as infection)

6.   How would Nancy's glucose of 704 be treated?
       Initially, she will be treated with an IV insulin drip. Subcutaneous insulin is not appropriate at this time because it is slower to act and is absorbed slower due to decreased fluid volume and poor tissue perfusion. Only regular insulin is administered IV. It is fast acting, and when given IV, it peaks in 30 - 60 minutes.

7.   The House Officer (HO) does not order $NaHCO_3$ for Nancy's pH of 7.0, would you remind her to?
       No. As glucose and fluids are administered, acidosis will correct itself. Use of sodium bicarbonate is often avoided since the acidosis is self-limiting and rebound alkalosis from too much bicarbonate is also to be avoided.

8.   The HO orders "KCl 20 mEq X 2 doses over 1 hour each, to begin in 3 hours". But her admission K was 6.2. Would you question this order?
       No. Metabolic acidosis causes potassium to move out of the cells and into the serum. Therefore, serum potassium will increase but intracellular potassium is decreased. Osmotic diuresis causes potassium to be lost in the urine. When insulin is administered, potassium is transported back into the cells with the glucose causing a decrease in serum potassium. Will usually see a decrease in serum potassium within the first 1-4 hours following initiation of therapy. Potassium therapy is started once serum potassium falls to about 5. K-Phos may also be ordered, as phosphorus is also decreased due to osmotic diuresis.

9.   What is the IVF you should hang for Ms. NPH?
       Normal saline. Sodium is lost with osmotic diuresis.

10.   Nancy's BP was 80/40 on admission. The admission orders contain an order for Dopamine 12 mcg/kg/minute. Would you question this order?
       Yes. Her low blood pressure is due to hypovolemia and the treatment of choice is fluid resuscitation. Vasopressors are used for those patients whose BP does not respond to the fluid increase.

Case C: Beau Jones

Beau Jones, a frail appearing 78 year old nursing home patient, is transferred to your hospital with the following history:

He is a Type II diabetic who has been diet controlled for five years. Four days ago, he developed flu-like symptoms, becoming very nauseated and was unable to take food or fluids. His physician ordered a high carbohydrate tube feeding to be initiated to prevent malnutrition and dehydration. Two days ago, the nurses noted that Mr. Jones had developed a decreased level of consciousness which has been progressively worsening. On admission to the hospital, Beau does not respond to anything but deep pain stimulation. His vital signs are as follows:

BP = 88/48, P = 126, R = 32 and shallow, T = 102

1. What available cues are there that would suggest that Beau is experiencing a diabetic crisis?
History of Type II diabetes, diet controlled. He has been not been taking food or fluids for several days. High carbohydrate diet has been given. Decreased level of consciousness.

2. Based on his clinical presentation AND history, what is probably his medical diagnosis?
DKA: _____
HHNC: __X__
Hypoglycemic Coma: _____

3. What labs would be helpful in confirming this diagnosis and what findings would be expected? (Compare how the results would differ, based on each diagnosis)

Laboratory Data	DKA	HHNC
Serum Glucose	*>300 - 800 mg/dL*	*600 - 2,500 mg/dL*
Anion Gap	*Positive (> 7 mEq/L)*	*Negative (<7 mEq/L)*
Serum ketones	*Positive*	*Absent*
Serum osmolality	*<330 mOsm/L*	*>330 mOsm/L*
Serum pH	*<7.30,*	*≥7.30,*
HCO₃	*≤ 15 mEq/L*	*≥ 15 mEq/L*

[For more comparisons of DKA to HHNC please refer to Table 24-5]]

4. What other signs and symptoms would you anticipate related to his probable diagnosis?
Slow, insidious onset. Profound dehydration and hypovolemic shock signs and symptoms. No ketone breath, no Kussmaul's breathing.

5. What would be your PRIORITY nursing diagnoses based on this diagnosis? What expected patient outcomes will you evaluate? What PRIORITY nursing interventions would be appropriate during his crisis state?

#1 Nursing Diagnosis: *Fluid volume deficit r/t severe osmotic diuresis*
EPOs:
1) *I = O*
2) *SBP = within normal range for patient (specify)*
3) *U/O = >30 mL/Hr*
4) *Normal skin turgor*
5) *Usual mental status*
6) *BUN and creatinine WNL*

Priority Nursing Intervention(s):
1) *Monitor for clinical manifestations of fluid volume deficit, report abnormals*

> *2)* *Monitor hemodynamic status, as available*
> *3)* *Monitor laboratory tests as ordered, report abnormals*

#2 Nursing Diagnosis: *Pot. for injury r/t electrolyte imbalances secondary to osmotic diuresis*
EPOs:
1) *Serum electrolytes within normal limits*
2) *Usual cardiac rhythm*
3) *ABG within acceptable ranges*

Priority Nursing Intervention(s):
1) *Assess for the clinical manifestations of electrolyte imbalances (esp. potassium and sodium)*
2) *Replace electrolytes as ordered.*
3) *Monitor for therapeutic and nontherapeutic effects of drug therapy.*

#3 Nursing Diagnosis: *Alt. in nutrition: less than body requirements*
EPOs:
1) *Serum glucose within acceptable range*
2) *Negative serum and urine ketones*

Priority Nursing Interventions(s):
1) *Monitor for therapeutic and nontherapeutic effects of insulin therapy*
2) *Monitor serum glucose, ketones, as ordered and report abnormals*
3) *Monitor daily intake closely*

****

6. What population is at particular risk for development of HHNC?

The classic HHNC patient is an elderly, Type II diabetic who is infirm. The individual is often institutionalized. The HHNC episode is generally triggered by an acute physiologic stress.

7. What is the pathological basis for HHNC?

Insufficient insulin is available to be able to cover increased glucose levels caused by a physiologic stress. As glucose rises → increased glucosuria → osmotic diuresis with loss of Na, K, Phos- → to dehydration occurs and patient becomes increasingly hyperosmolar. Once set into motion, the pathologic process is the same as DKA with the exception of no ketoacidosis. It is believed that ketoacidosis is avoided in HHNC because there is sufficient insulin being secreted to prevent breakdown of fatty acids to ketones.

Case Studies
Immunocompetence

Case A: The Case of Mrs. Quinn

SITUATION:

Mrs. Quinn, 42 years old, was admitted to your hospital floor with an acute urinary tract infection. At admission, she was complaining of nausea and begins vomiting, which has worsened over the past 24 hours. Her vital signs on admission were:

BP = 96/58, HR = 115/minute, RR = 20/minute, temp. = 103.8 F (o)

Her medical history includes previous U.T.I.s over the past several years. She is allergic to IVP dye and Penicillin.

Admission Orders:

IV D_5 0.45 NS at 100 mL/hour

Tylenol 650 mg (PO0 every 4 hours PRN elevated temperature

Pain control: Demerol 50 mg with Phenergan 25 mg (IM) every 4 hours PRN

Diet: NPO until nausea ceases

Cephradine 1 gm (IV) q 6 hours

Four Hours Post-Admission

You are the evening nurse who is taking over care of Mrs. Quinn. At 1800, you administer the ordered IV Cephradine, which infused in over 30 minutes. At 1845, Mrs. Quinn's son comes up to the nurses' station and tells you that something is wrong with his mother.

Upon entering the room, you note the following: Mrs. Quinn has facial edema and a maculopapular rash. She is scratching her skin and complaining of severe itching. You take her vital signs and obtain a BP of 152/88, HR of 126/minute, and RR of 32/minute.

1. What type of immune response is Mrs. Quinn's clinical presentation suggestive of?

2. What is the pathophysiologic basis of what has occurred?

3. What are the correct INITIAL nursing responses to Mrs. Quinn's situation?

4. What are your priority nursing diagnoses expected patient outcomes (EPOs) and interventions?

5.   What type of drug therapy is the physician likely to order?

6.   What other physician orders might be ordered to support Mrs. Quinn during her acute phase of the reaction?

7.   How could this situation have been avoided?

Case B: The Case of Mark Y

SITUATION

Mark Y. is a 33 year old business man who was admitted to the hospital with a diagnosis of hepatic failure. He presents with the following history.

Mark has been ill for approximately six weeks. He has a ten pound weight loss though he denies nausea, vomiting, or diarrhea. His admission vital signs were: BP = 110/80, HR = 140, RR = 32, Temp = 105.5 F (o). He has a nonproductive cough with diminished left lower lobe breath sounds. He was diagnosed with Hepatitis B last week by a private physician.

Admission Labs:

CBC with differential count:

WBC	=	3.1			
Hgb	=	7.7			
Hct	=	21.5			
Platelets	=	50,000			
Lymphs	=	20			
Monos	=	9			

PT	=	19.2 / 12.0

Electrolytes:

Na	=	125
K	=	4.5
Albumin	=	1.8
Total Protein	=	4.6

AST	=	361
ALT	=	271
LDH	=	559

B cell	=	98	(Nl = 70 - 816)
T cell	=	205	(Nl = 750 - 4,368)

1. Assess Mr. Y's humoral immunity status:

2. Assess Mr. Y's cellular immunity status:

3. Assess Mr. Y's hematologic status:

4. Assess Mr. Y's nutritional status:

5. What opportunistic infections is Mr. Young at risk for contracting? What assessment data would be suggestive of these diseases?

6. What diagnostic tests are confirmatory for AIDS?

7. How does AIDS affect the immune system?

8. What nursing diagnoses would be appropriate for Mr. Y? State expected patient outcomes for each diagnosis:

Nursing Diagnosis	Expected Patient Outcomes
1)	
2)	
3)	
4)	

Case C: The Case of Anne Baker

SITUATION:
Ann Baker is a 28 year old woman who is admitted with a history of systemic lupus erythematosis (SLE), acute exacerbation. She has a history of depression and a previous suicide attempt. She has severe left hip pain. Ms. Baker has had a 15 pound weight gain in the last 3 weeks. Current medications include:
   Ibuprofen 800 mg TID (PO)
   Prednisone 15 mg QD (PO)

1. SLE is an autoimmune disease. How does this differ from a disease process such as AIDS?

2. What type of laboratory tests are used to diagnose autoimmune diseases?

3. What impact would her current medications have on her immune system?

4. What are appropriate nursing diagnoses for Ms. Baker? How do these diagnoses compare with common nursing diagnoses associated with AIDS?

Case D: The Case of Andy W.

SITUATION:
Andy Wade was diagnosed with glomerulonephritis 5 years ago. He recently required hospitalization for treatment of hypertension and anemia. At that time, an AV fistula was placed and he has been on dialysis three time per week. He is admitted presently for a renal transplant from his brother. Preoperatively, he is receiving methylprednisolone, antithymocyte globulin, and azathioprine.

1. What action do these medications have on the immune system?

2. Mr. Wade receives the transplant. What assessment data would indicate that he is rejecting the transplant?

3. What medications may Mr. Wade receive to counteract the rejection? How do these medications affect the immune system?

4. What nursing diagnoses would be appropriate for Mr. Wade related to these medications?

Case Studies
Immunocompetence
Instructor Guide

Case A: The Case of Mrs. Quinn

SITUATION:

Mrs. Quinn, 42 years old, was admitted to your hospital floor with an acute urinary tract infection (UTI). At admission, she was complaining of nausea and begins vomiting, which has worsened over the past 24 hours. Her vital signs on admission were:

BP = 96/58, HR = 115/minute, RR = 20/minute, temp. = 103.8 F (o)

Her medical history includes previous UTIs over the past several years. She is allergic to IVP dye and Penicillin.

Admission Orders:

IV D$_5$0.45 NS at 100 mL/hour

Tylenol 650 mg (PO0 every 4 hours PRN elevated temperature

Pain control: Demerol 50 mg with Phenergan 25 mg (IM) every 4 hours PRN

Diet: NPO until nausea ceases

Cephradine 1 gm (IV) q 6 hours

Four Hours Post-Admission

You are the evening nurse who is taking over care of Mrs. Quinn. At 1800, you administer the ordered IV Cephradine, which infused in over 30 minutes. At 1845, Mrs. Quinn's son comes up to the nurses' station and tells you that something is wrong with his mother.

Upon entering the room, you not the following: Mrs. Quinn has facial edema and a maculopapular rash. She is scratching her skin and complaining of severe itching. You take her vital signs and obtain a BP of 152/88, HR of 126/minute, and RR of 32/minute.

1. What type of immune response is Mrs. Quinn's clinical presentation suggestive of?
    A type II hypersensitivity response

2. What is the pathophysiologic basis of what has occurred?
    IgM and IgG react directly with cell surface antigens, activating the complement system and producing direct injury to the cell surface. In a transfusion reaction, RBC surfaces are damaged by antibodies and the cell is destroyed.

3. What are the correct INITIAL nursing responses to Mrs. Quinn's situation?
    a. *Stop the antibiotic infusion. Disconnect IV tubing at the catheter site. Infuse D$_5$W. Be prepared to support the patient's cardiac and/or pulmonary status should they become compromised. (Blood pressure can drop rapidly if reaction is severe)*
    b. *Call the physician*

4. What are your priority nursing diagnoses expected patient outcomes (EPOs) and interventions?
    a. *High risk for ineffective airway clearance r/t airway edema associated with anaphylactic reaction*
    b. *High risk for decreased cardiac output r/t cardiovascular collapse associated with anaphylactic reaction*

5. What type of drug therapy is the physician likely to order?
    Primary treatment: antihistamine (e.g., Benadryl); epinephrine
    Other: Aminophylline, steroid therapy

6.   What other physician orders might be ordered to support Mrs. Quinn during her acute phase of the reaction?

Oxygen therapy if necessary. Blood pressure support by vasoconstriction or fluid resuscitation.

7.   How could this situation have been avoided?

The nurse should have questioned the Cephradine order since there is a positive history of penicillin allergy.

Case B: The Case of Mark Y

SITUATION

Mark Y. is a 33 year old business man who was admitted to the hospital with a diagnosis of hepatic failure. He presents with the following history.

Mark has been ill for approximately six weeks. He has a ten pound weight loss though he denies nausea, vomiting, or diarrhea. His admission vital signs were: BP = 110/80, HR = 140, RR = 32, Temp = 105.5 F (o). He has a nonproductive cough with diminished left lower lobe breath sounds. He was diagnosed with Hepatitis B last week by a private physician. He tested seropositive for HIV 5 years ago.

Admission Labs:

CBC with differential count:			PT	=	19.2 / 12.0	
WBC	=	3.1	Electrolytes:			
Hgb	=	7.7	Na	=	125	
Hct	=	21.5	K	=	4.5	
Platelets =		50,000	Albumin	=	1.8	
Lymphs =		20%	Total Protein	=	4.6	
Monos = ·		9				
AST	=	361	B cell	=	98	(Nl = 70 - 816)
ALT	=	271	T cell	=	205	(Nl = 750 - 4,368)
LDH	=	559				

1. Assess Mr. Y's humoral immunity status:
   B cells are OK; WBC = decreased. Monos = Increased (indicative of chronic infection). These are nonspecific immune responses. Mark is still able to mobilize a fever response.

2. Assess Mr. Y's cellular immunity status:
   T Cells are decreased and WBC is decreased

3. Assess Mr. Y's hematologic status:
   Decrease platelets, increased PT = places his at increased risk for bleeding
   WBC and lymphocyte count = low; low TLC – is at high risk for infection
   Hgb and Hct are both decreased = potential for decreased tissue oxygenation

4. Assess Mr. Y's nutritional status:
   His albumin and protein levels are low. His protein electrophoresis would be nice to see to evaluate gamma globulins.

5. What opportunistic infections is Mr. Young at risk for contracting? What assessment data would be suggestive of these diseases?
   PCP, CMV, herpes, Cryptococcal pneumoccal infections
   S/S: mental status changes, vision changes, cough, skin lesions, vasodilation, fever

6. What diagnostic tests are CONFIRMATORY for AIDS: *ELISA and Western Blot Test*

7. How does HIV affect the immune system?
   HIV doesn't cause the primary disease. It causes a decrease in Helper T-cells and Killer T cells and an increase in Suppressor T cells.

8. What nursing diagnoses would be appropriate for Mr. Y?

> *Impaired gas exchange*
> *Impaired skin integrity*
> *High risk for fluid volume deficit*
> *Alt. nutrition: less than body requirements*
> *Infection*
> *Anticipatory grieving*

Case C: The Case of Anne Baker

SITUATION:

Ann Baker is a 28 year old woman who is admitted with a history of systemic lupus erythematosis (SLE), acute exacerbation. She has a history of depression and a previous suicide attempt. She has severe left hip pain. Ms. Baker has had a 15 pound weight gain in the last 3 weeks. Current medications include:

Ibuprofen 800 mg TID (PO)

Prednisone 15 mg QD (PO)

1. SLE is an autoimmune disease. How does this differ from a disease process such as AIDS?
   1) *No external etiology*
   2) *Immuosuppression is not the problem, rather, over-work of the immune system*
   3) *Decrease incidence of opportunistic infections and illness related to the primary disease*

2. What type of laboratory tests are used to diagnose autoimmune diseases?
   Immunoglobulins, C Reactive Proteins, Protein electrophoresis, LE Prep, ANA, ESR

3. What impact would her current medications have on her immune system?
   1) ***Ibuprofen – nonsteroidal antiinflammatory***
   2) ***Prednisone – steroid, antiinflammatory***
   Both calm the inflammatory process down, reducing the autoimmune inflammatory symptoms

4. What are appropriate nursing diagnoses for Ms. Baker? How do these diagnoses compare with common nursing diagnoses associated with AIDS?
   Pain
   Impaired physical mobility
   Alt. in tissue perfusion
   The high risk for injury r/t infection is not generally associated with SLE unless it is a complication of steroid therapy.

Case D: The Case of Andy W.

SITUATION:
Andy Wade was diagnosed with glomerulonephritis 5 years ago. He recently required hospitalization for treatment of hypertension and anemia. At that time, an AV fistula was placed and he has been on dialysis three time per week. He is admitted presently for a renal transplant from his brother. Preoperatively, he is receiving methylprednisolone, antithymocyte globulin, and azathioprine.

1. What action do these medications have on the immune system?
    Methylprednisolone: *antiinflammatory activity*
    Antithymocyte globulin: *decreased T cells*
    Antithymocyte globulin: *Decreased T cells*
    Azathioprine (Imuran): *Decreased lymphocyte activity*

2. Mr. Wade receives the transplant. What assessment data would indicate that he is rejecting the transplant?
    Decreased urine output, rapid weight gain, BUN and creatinine increase, hypertension, fever, increased WBC (both fever and WBC count will depend on level of immunosuppression)

3. What medications may Mr. Wade receive to counteract the rejection? How do these medications affect the immune system?
    OKT-3 (murine antihuman mature antibody T cell) reacts with and blocks the function of T cells
    Steroid Therapy: Antiinflammatory activity decreases phagocytosis
    Cyclosporine (Sandimmune): suppresses humoral immunity and cell mediated response so there is a decrease in B cells.

4. What nursing diagnoses would be appropriate for Mr. Wade related to these medications?
    Infection
    Fluid volume excess
    Fear r/t organ rejection
    Guilt r/t donation

Case Study
The Case of Joan T.

[This is a complex patient case study. It has multisystem implications and a rich database that would lend itself well to clinical investigation in multiple topic areas]

The Patient: Joan T, 54 years old.

The Admission Diagnosis: Pancreatitis, urinary tract infection, and clinical dehydration.

Past History:

Joan has a history of rheumatoid arthritis, polymyositis, hypertension, and Raynaud's Syndrome. Five years ago, she was diagnosed with mild liver disease, specifically, chronic persistent cirrhosis. Her surgical history includes a partial hysterectomy with a cystocele repair, and cholecystectomy. She does not drink any alcoholic beverages but has a history of smoking ½ PPD for 30 years.

Medication History:

Prednisone 10 mg QD for 6 years
Zantac 150 mg q HS
Bactrim 160 mg BID
Atenecol 100 mg BID
Ibuprofen 600 mg q 6 h PRN

Recent History:

Joan was brought into the Emergency Department with complaints of increasingly severe abdominal pain and nausea and vomiting over a 1 ½ week period. She has been attempting to sip liquids but vomits it up with one-half hour after drinking. She states that her urine has been intermittently. She denies fever, cough, dysuria or chest pain. Her last bowel movement was three days before admission. She has lost approximately 10 pounds over the two week period prior to admission. Her admission vital signs were as follows:

BP = 149/94, HR = 83/minute, RR = 24/minute, Temp = 97.8 F

Hospitalization Course

Three days following admission, Joan developed an acute GI bleed with a significant drop of Hct from 29.1 at admission to 15. An emergent endoscopy confirmed a duodenal ulcer and upper GI bleeding. The ulcer was given sclerosant injection therapy during the endoscopy. The bleeding was successfully halted. At that time she had an NG tube placed, her Motrin was discontinued, she was made NPO, a PT and PTT were drawn STAT, and she received 4 units of packed RBCs and 2 liters of IV fluids. Prior to treatment, she had a large, black, loose stool. Her blood pressure was 110/70 and pulse was 70/minute (while receiving Atenolol).

One week later, she developed bilateral lower extremity deep vein thromboses and subsequently had an intravascular filter placed to prevent emboli complications. Several days later, she received a vagotomy and pyloroplasty and was admitted to the Surgical ICU following surgery. In the SICU she required mechanical ventilatory support, antibiotic therapy, and antihypertensives. Several days after transfer to the SICU she sustained a left lower lung collapse, which was confirmed by portable chest x-ray. The x-ray also showed evidence of mild pulmonary edema. Currently, she remains in the SICU with a tracheostomy and she is ventilator dependent.

Initial Chart Notations:

Labs: (See #1 Column in table)
Urine : U/A = 4+ bacteria, increased WBC
Pain: Dull, throbbing pain
Abdomen:
Soft, + bowel sounds, tender epigastrum (RUQ > RLQ), No rebound or guarding

Pulmonary
Right posterior basilar crackles

General Appearance
Cushinoid features, with mood face. Ecchymoses noted on chest. Skin is thin and translucent.

Laboratory Trends

Test	#1 (3/26)	#2 (3/29)	#3 (3/31)	#4 (4/16)
Na	135			142
K	3.6			3.5
Cl	110			112
Ca (Total)	4.5			3.7
Ca (Ion)				2.31
WBC	6.4			12.4
Lymphocytes				2%
Hgb				10.7
Hct	29.1	15.1		31.6
PT	12			12.5
PTT	27.3			28.6
Platelets	152			96
AST	31	22		
ALT	33	24		
LDH	304	662		
CPK	17	26		
Alk. Phos.	71	50		
Protein	6.1	4.8		
Albumin	3.2	2.8		
Bilirubin	0.2	0.4		
BUN	20			
Creatinine	1.0			
Amylase	109	94	383	246
Lipase	600	1629	2262	2236

Additional Data (of optional nutritional interest)

Oxygen Consumption Study
Temp = 97.9, P = 72, $ - 28, BP 150/100
Patient quiet; Present nutrition: TPN @ 65 mL/hr; 20% lipids (250 cc)
Indirect Calorimetry:
Measured Energy Expenditure (MEE) = 1330 calories
Predicted Energy Expenditure (PEE) = 1190 calories
Respiratory Quotient = 0.95
MEE / PEE Ratio = 1.12
O_2 consumption = 126 mL/min/m^2. CO_2 production = 119 mL/min/m^2

Most Current Data

An ultrasound of the abdomen had the following results: No biliary ductal dilatation; liver has normal appearance; mild fatty infiltration of pancreas.

Neurological:
Oriented to person, place and time. Writes coherent notes to staff and husband

Pulmonary:

Loud rhonchi in right and left upper lobe and left lower lobe; crackles heard

#8 Shiley tracheostomy in place

On mechanical ventilator on Assist/Control at rate of 12 (over-breathing @ 15/min.), FiO_2 40%, TV 700 mL, PEEP 10 cm H_2O

ABG = pH 7.5, $PaCO_2$ = 35, PaO_2 = 76, HCO_3 = 29

Suctioning for thick, plugs with small amount of bloody content

Chest x-ray: mild pulmonary edema

Cardiovascular:

CVP = 15 - 16

BP 149/94

ECG = sinus tachycardia

Auscultated: S1 and S2, no murmur

Abdominal:

Abdomen distended and firm

Bowel sounds hypoactive in all 4 quadrants

Gastric secretions: Guaiac = +

Integumentary:

Generalized ecchymosis

Pitting edema in LUE and BLE

Sanguineous drainage from midline abdominal incision

Stage I decubitus on coccyx

Multiple skin tears noted

Compression stockings on BLE

Tracheostomy site is red, with ecchymoses present

Arterial line in place in left radial artery. Attached to direct BP measurement monitor

Renal:

Foley catheter in place

Output = 2450 mL,

Fluid Balance:

24 hours -- Intake = 3334 mL with Output 2,450 mL

4 day total – Intake = 13,000 mL; Output = 7,255 mL

Weight Trends:

On admission: 132 pounds

Current: 145 pounds

Vital Signs Ranges:

BP   101/66 - 165/94;   HR   104 - 125;   RR   14/12 - 21/12

MAP   78 - 115

Comfort:

Rates pain at 5 on a 10 point scale

Facial grimaces when doing passive ROM exercises, turning and transfer into chair (BP and HR also increase)

Receiving PCA analgesia of demerol – forgets to push button or doses off

Current Medications:

Metoprolol 5mg (IV)	Hydrocortisone 50 mg (IV) BID
Heparin 5000 units (SQ) BID	Piperacillin 1 Gm/2.5 mL (IV) q 6 hours
Nystatin 5 mL (PO) TID	Lipids 20% 500 mL over 12 hours
Nifedipine 10 mg (SL) q 4 hours	Gentamycin 150 mg (IV) q 24 hours
Vancomycin 850 mg (IV) q 36 hours	Acetaminophen 650 mg (PR) q 4 hours
Diphenhydramine 50 mg (PO) QD	Cimetidine 300 mg (IV) q 6 hours

The Case of Joan T Study Guide

(Instructor: This is a complex patient with multiple problems. Her data can support multiple approaches for study. His particular Study Guide focuses on her pancreatic problem)

1. What risk factors, if any, does Joan have for developing pancreatitis? (look at Table 25-3: Major Etiology of Acute Pancreatitis)

    She has none of the common risk factors. The drug related connection is the closest. In the actual case, the origin of the pancreatitis was never found. It was decided that it most likely resulted from her long term steroid therapy, or possibly her duodenal ulcer impinging on the pancreas, or triglyceridemia.

2. Examine her labs. What laboratory trends would you expect to find ($\uparrow$, $\downarrow$, $\leftrightarrow$). What are her own trends? Do her own trends support it?

Test	Typical Trend	Joan's Trends
Amylase	$\uparrow\uparrow$	$\uparrow$
Lipase	$\uparrow$	$\uparrow\uparrow$
Glucose	$\uparrow$	$\leftrightarrow$
Calcium	$\downarrow$	$\downarrow$
WBC	$\uparrow$	$\uparrow$
BUN	$\uparrow$	$\leftrightarrow$
LDH	$\uparrow$	$\uparrow$
AST	$\uparrow\uparrow$	$\leftrightarrow$
Albumin	$\downarrow$	$\downarrow$
PaO_2	$\downarrow$	$\downarrow$

    Overall, her labs were quite consistent with the "typical" picture except for her AST and BUN, levels, which did not elevate.

3. Examine the Ransom Criteria (Table 25-5). How many of the criteria does she have? What is her mortality risk based on the criteria? *She has at least 4. Her mortality risk would be at 15%*

4. The table below lists common clinical findings consistent with acute pancreatitis. Examine her actual clinical presentation and indicate whether or not she displayed the various findings.

Manifestations	Joan's Manifestations
Gastrointestinal • Anorexia • Upper GI tenderness without rigidity • Abdominal distention • Steatorrhea • Diarrhea • Peritoneal Signs • $\downarrow$ or no bowel sounds • $\uparrow$ abdominal pain • abdom. rigidity, guarding, rebound tenderness, leukocytosis, tachycardia, fever	*Joan had problems with nausea and vomiting, can occur. She had upper GI tenderness without rigidity. Her abdomen was distended. She had decreased bowel sounds and increased abdominal pain.*
Integumentary • Cullen's sign • Grey Turner's sign	*No data*

Manifestations	Joan's Manifestations
Cardiopulmonary • Decreased BP • Tachycardia • Pleural effusion - adventitious breath sounds , particularly crackles • Pulmonary edema • Respiratory insufficiency / failure • Pneumonia	*She had a labile blood pressure and tachycardia. She had adventitious breath sounds and mild pulmonary edema. She required mechanical ventilation for respiratory problems.*
Electrolyte Imbalances • Chvostek's sign • Trousseau's sign	*These were not performed*

5. Examine Joan's medical management. What interventions are consistent with typical supportive therapy?

Support Medical Management	Joan's Medical Management
Hemodynamic Support	*Joan did not develop a hemodynamic crisis. She was adequately supported by fluid resuscitation. She was monitored closely using CVP measurement and arterial line direct BP readings.*
Fluid Resuscitation	*Joan did receive fluid resuscitation – however, it was not needed for treatment of her pancreatitis, which was not hemorrhagic. She required it to treat her GI hemorrhage from a duodenal ulcer.*
Inotropes	*She did not require*
Oxygenation Support	*Joan did require support of oxygenation and ventilation. Her pulmonary situation was complicated by her long history of smoking. She became ventilator dependent. She required frequent suctioning.*
Renal	*Her renal function did not become compromised, and did not require specific therapy. Her output was strictly monitored.*
Nutritional	*She received nutritional support fluids to prevent stimulation of the GI tract to allow the pancreas to rest: TPN at 65 mL/hr and 20% lipids.*
Pain Control	*She was on a PCA pump, using Demerol. Demerol is the drug of choice in acute pancreatitis. Morphine is often avoided because it can cause spasms of the sphincter of Oddi.*
Infection	*Joan was placed on several IV antibiotics. She was admitted with a UTI and was at risk for developing other infections*

6. Based on Joan's hospital course, list nursing diagnoses that would be appropriate:
(Instructor, the following is only a partial list of some of the most obvious ones)
Pain: epigastric / abdominal
Altered nutrition: less than body requirements
Ineffective breathing pattern
Altered comfort: nausea and vomiting
Infection
High risk for decreased cardiac output r/t GI hemorrhage

Case Study
The Case of C.R. Cramer

On the third of March of this year, Mr. C.R. Cramer, a 50 year old store owner and farmer was admitted to your unit from an outlying hospital with a diagnosis of tetanus. Six days prior to admission, he stepped on a nail. Rather than seeking medical attention, he cleaned the wound and continued to work. At day #4 post-injury, he noted slight weakness/stiffness in his legs and tightness of his jaw. By Day #6, he asked to be taken to the local emergency department. At that time, his joints were very stiff and he could no longer open his mouth. He was rapidly transferred to this regional medical center in mild respiratory distress. His neuromuscular status steadily deteriorated, requiring mechanical ventilation. He also required amputation of his injured right leg due to an extensive infective process.

Relevant History
C.R. has a 5 year history of non-insulin dependent diabetes mellitus which has been diet controlled. His history also includes a myocardial infarction (MI) one year ago, one episode of congestive heart failure, and arthritis. He has a 22 year history of smoking one pack of cigarettes per day. He is allergic to Penicillin.

Systematic Assessment:
Height/Weight: C.R. is 6 foot, 1 inch tall. Usual weight = 210 pounds, large framed.

Neurologic: Currently he is receiving Norcuron, a neuromuscular blockade drug, which has completely paralyzed him. You are unable to assess his neurologic status at this time.

Respiratory: He is on a Bear V mechanical ventilator. A chest x-ray shows right lower lobe (RLL) pneumonia. He has empyema in his RLL. The pneumonia is diagnosed as pseudomonas. You are able to auscultate scattered rhonchi throughout his lung fields with decreased sounds evident in the bases, particularly on the right side. He is requiring endotracheal suctioning every hour for moderate to large amounts of green foul smelling sputum.

Cardiac: Heart sounds = S_1 and S_2 auscultated. No murmur is noted.

Integumentary: A small decubitus is noted on his coccyx. His oral mucous membranes have white patches which are suspicious of a yeast infection.

Musculoskeletal: Extensive contractures are noted. You also note that he has a right below the knee amputation (BKA). The flap shows evidence of probable yeast infection.

Gastrointestinal: His abdomen is slightly distended. He has diminished bowel sounds in all four quadrants. His latest stool guaiacs are positive.

Genitourinary: A foley catheter is in place. His urine output has been consistently >30 mL/Hr. His urine appears yellow and slightly cloudy.

Vital Signs: BP = 164/90, P = 108, R = per ventilator, T = 101-102 peaks

Physicians Orders:
C.R.'s admission orders:
> 5% Dextrose and Normal Saline with 20 mEq potassium chloride at 100 mL/Hr.
> Heparin Drip of 1,000 units per hour
> Versed Drip at 8 mg/Hr.
> Insulin per sliding scale
> Albuterol nebulizer treatments every 6 hours (2 puffs/treatment)
> Nystatin 15mL swish/spit every 4 hours
> Nystatin powder to stump every 6 hours
> IV antibiotic order
> STAT CBC with differential and serum albumin

C.R's nutrition orders 7 days after admission:
> Insert small bore enteric feeding tube per routine.
> Portable abdominal x-ray 24 hours following enteric tube placement to verify location of tip.
> If placement is verified, initiate Osmolyte HN @ 25mL/hr and increase rate by 25mL/hr every 4 hours if tolerated to final rate of 100mL/hr.
> Obtain a urine urea nitrogen/nitrogen intake balance.

Dietary History

Mr. Cramer is a single man who lives alone. His closest relatives are two cousins who see him about once per week. They can only tell you that he is usually a good eater but does not watch what he eats very well to control his diabetes. They also tell you that he had a loss of appetite that increased steadily because he "felt so poorly" following his foot injury. No other diet history is available.

Summary of Significant Laboratory Results

White Blood Cell Count and Lymphocytes

	WBC	Lymphocytes
#1: At time of admission:	18,200	9.9%
#2: Midway into admission:	15,500	8.3%
#3: Most current:	10,200	7.3%

Serum Albumin

#1: At time of admission:	3.5 mg/dL
#2: Midway into admission:	3.0 mg/dL
#3: Most current:	1.8 mg/dL

Serum Prealbumin

#1: At time of admission:	No data
#2: Midway into admission:	21 mg/dL
#3: Most current:	16 mg/dL

Creatinine Height Index

#1: At time of admission:	No data
#2: Midway into admission:	73 %
#3: Most current:	65%

Nitrogen Balance Measurements

24 hour nitrogen intake:	54.3 g/24 hrs. (Nl intake = 56g/24 hrs.)
24 hour nitrogen excretion:	62.1 g/24 hrs.

Anthrometric Measurements

Mid-arm circumference:	On admission =	28.4 cm
	Current =	26.2cm

Serial Weights

Preadmission: 210 pounds
3/7 = 208, 3/9 = 203, 3/11 = 200, 3/13 = 195.6, 3/15 = 194, 3/17 = 191, 3/19 = 188, 3/21 = 186, 3/24 = 184

Your latest assessment

The date is 3/24. You have just completed your assessment. Significant findings included:

Neurologic: No change. He continues on a Norcuron drip. He is intermittently brought out from under the drip to check his neurologic status. During these periods, you note spastic limb activity and risus sardonicus. He is able to follow you with his eyes.

Respiratory: A chest tube is in place. You note a small amount of serous drainage. Scattered rhonchi are auscultated and his lung bases are both very diminished.

Cardiovascular: S_1 and S_2 are auscultated. 2+ to 3+ pitting peripheral edema.

Gastrointestinal: He continues on tube feedings at 100 mL/hr. He has hyperactive bowel sounds in all four quadrants. A rectal bag is in place to protect his skin from frequent diarrhea stools.

Genitourinary: A foley catheter is in place. His urine output remains > 30mL/hr.
Integumentary: His skin is very dry and is shedding. You note that his flesh is beginning to hang on his frame.

Musculoskeletal: His stump has several open lesions on it with an increase in drainage. A culture was taken of the lesions -- they were positive for candida albicans.

Vital Signs: BP = 108/64, P = 106, R = per ventilator, T = 100.6

The Case of C.R. Cramer Study Guide

Recent History/Reason for admission hospital:

Any factors present in history that might influence nutritional status?

Nutritional Assessment:
A. **Dietary History**
    1.   Pre-existing nutritional status (if available):

    2.   Calorie Count results (if available via dietary consultation):

    3.   Length of time patient on NPO status (prior to initiation of TPN, intralipids, tube feedings):

    4.   Nutritional Orders:

        TPN:

        Intralipids:

        Tube Feedings:

        Vitamin and/or mineral supplements:

        P.O. Diet:

B. **Nitrogen Balance**
    1.   Urine Urea Nitrogen (UUN) results (if available):
    2.   Has nitrogen balance been calculated? If yes, what were the results?
    3.   Anthrometric Measurements:
        1.   Pt. Height:_____
        2.   Pt. Weight: Include trends (admission → current):

            _____, _____, _____, _____, _____, _____

        3.   What is the total gain or loss of weight since admission?

        4.   Has the patient recently lost $\geq$10% of usual body weight?

        5.   Where does this patient fall on the 1983 Metropolitan Height & Weight Table?
            At admission: Above nl?___, Normal?___, Below nl?___.
            Currently: Above nl?___, Normal?___, Below nl?___.

6.   If this patient is obese, what should the ideal weight be? (This is important to consider for nutritional needs and drug dosage needs)

7.   Midarm Circumference (Refer to Table: Midarm Muscle Circumference)

      a.   Measure circumference 1/2 way between top of shoulder and elbow: _____.

      b.   Where does this patient's measurement fall according to the chart?
              Below 50% measurement?
              Above 50% measurement?

Midarm Muscle Circumference (50th Percentile)
Males: 45-54 = 28.2 55-64 = 27.8 65-74 = 26.8 Adapted from Bishop CW, et al: norms for Nutritional Assessment of American Adults for Upper Arm Anthropometry. Am J Clin Nutr 34 (11): 2530-2539, 1981

D.   Protein Measurements
1.   Visceral Protein
      a.   Serum Albumin (nl = $\geq$3.5 g/dL):

      b.   This patient's albumin trends over time:
              _____, _____, _____, _____

E.   Physical Assessment for Protein and Protein-Calorie Malnutrition:

1. Examine C.R.'s assessment data complete the following chart:

System	Presence (Yes/No)

1. Integumentary:
  -Decreased subcutaneous fat:
  -Flaky, dry skin:
  -Shedding of hair:

2. Musculoskeletal:
  -Muscle wasting:
  -Edema present:
3. Cardiovascular:
  -Evidence of decreased cardiac output

4. Evidence of lack of healing:

F.   What conclusions can you draw from the preceding nutritional data?

G.   What factors have contributed to his current nutritional status?

H.   Based on C.R.'s situation, what are the implications of waiting for a week or more before initiating nutritional support on this patient's status and prognosis?

I.   What nursing diagnoses would you apply to C.R.'s plan of care based on this nutritional status?

J.   What will be the focus of nursing management for C.R. related to his nutritional needs?

Checking C.R.'s Immunocompetence

1. **Total Lymphocyte Count (TLC)**

    a. Examine the CBC with differential at various points during C.R.'s hospitalization. Using the given formula, determine the TLC. What is the significance to this patient?

    $$TLC = \frac{\% \text{ Lymphocytes X WBC}}{100}$$

    > [exa: Pt. % lymphocytes = 10%. WBC = 10,000.
    > $$\frac{10.0 \text{ X } 10,000}{100} = 1,000]$$

    Early TLC:_____

    Mid-hospitalization TLC:_____

    Most current TLC:_____

    b. What do the above trends tell you about this patient's immunocompetence status?

2. Which of the following critical cues suggesting immunocompetence problems does C.R. exhibit, if any?

Critical Cue	Present (Y / N)
Fever	_____
Poor wound healing	_____
Abnormal CBC with Diff.	_____
Abnormal coagulation studies	_____
Recurrent, prolonged, or severe infections	_____
Secondary infections	_____
Immunosuppressive drug therapy	_____
Other at-risk factors	_____

3. Based on the available data relevant to C.R.'s nutrition and immune status, you would conclude that his immune status was:

The Case of C.R. Cramer Study Guide:
Instructor Guide

(Instructor Note: C.R. Cramer is a complex patient who developed complications from a tetanus episode. Of particular interest to this case is that he was clinically starved and had altered immunocompetency – therefor it fits very well for study of nutrition and immunocompetence. This case is also written as a Problem Solving Exercise)

Recent History/Reason for admission hospital:
>*Puncture wound via stepping on nail. Cleaned wound and did not seek medical treatment. Developed progressive weakness and stiffness in legs & tightness in jaw. By day #6 required hospitalization.*

Any factors present in history that might influence nutritional status?
>*non-insulin diabetic. Hx of CHF and MI.*

Nutritional Assessment:
A.   **Dietary History**
1.   Pre-existing nutritional status (if available):
>*Usually a "good eater" but doesn't watch his diet as he should. Family tells nurse that he has had decreased appetite for about one week prior to admission because he "felt so poorly".*

2.   Calorie Count results (if available via dietary consultation): ***Not available***

3.   Length of time patient on NPO status (prior to initiation of TPN, intralipids, tube feedings):
>*NPO for 7 days following admission*

4.   Nutritional Orders:

TPN: *None*
Intralipids: *None*
Tube Feedings: *Osmolyte HN @ 25 mL/hr & increase rate by 25 mL/hr every 4 hours if tol. to a final rate of 100 mL/hr.*
Vitamin and/or mineral supplements: *None*
P.O. Diet: *None*

B.   **Nitrogen Balance**
1.   Urine Urea Nitrogen (UUN) results (if available):
>*62.1 g/hr hours*
2.   Has nitrogen balance been calculated? If yes, what were the results?
>*Nitrogen intake measured at 54.3 g/24 hrs. Negative nitrogen balance of 7.8 g.*
3.   Anthrometric Measurements:
    1.   Pt. Height : *6 foot, 1 inch*

    2.   Pt. Weight: Include trends (admission ---> current):
    >*Admission: 210, 3/7 = 208, 3/11 = 200, 3/15 = 195, 3/19 = 188, 3/24 = 184*

    3.   What is the total gain or loss of weight since admission?
    >*26 pounds*

    4.   Has the patient recently lost ≥10% of usual body weight?
    >*Yes he has*
    5.   Where does this patient fall on the 1983 Metropolitan Height & Weight Table?
    At admission: Above nl? X , Normal?___, Below nl?___.

Currently: Above nl?___, Normal? _X_, Below nl?___.

6.   If this patient is obese, what should the ideal weight be? (This is important to consider for nutritional needs and drug dosage needs)
According to the Metropolitan chart, he should weigh160-174. This is figured based on his height, size of frame.

7.   Midarm Circumference (Refer to Table: Midarm Muscle Circumference)
   a.   Measure circumference 1/2 way between top of shoulder and elbow: **_28.4_**; on admission and **_27.3_** currently
   b.   Where does this patient's measurement fall according to the chart?
   Below 50% measurement?
   Above 50% measurement?
   On admission, he was above the 50 percentile. His latest measurement shows that he has fallen below the 50%.

Midarm Muscle Circumference (50th Percentile)
Males: 45-54 = 28.2 55-64 = 27.8 65-74 = 26.8 Adapted from Bishop CW, et al: norms for Nutritional Assessment of American Adults for Upper Arm Anthropometry. Am J Clin Nutr 34 (11): 2530-2539, 1981

D.   Protein Measurements
   1.   Visceral Protein
      a.   Serum Albumin (nl = $\geq$3.5 g/dL):
      1.8 mg/dL is the most current
      b.   This patient's albumin trends over time:
      Admission: 3.5 mg/dL, Midway into admission: 3.0, most current: 1.8

   2.   Total Lymphocyte Count (TLC)
      a.   Examine the CBC with differential at various points during the patient's hospitalization. Using the given formula, determine the TLC. What is the significance to this patient?

$$TLC = \frac{\% \text{ Lymphocytes X WBC}}{100}$$

[exa: Pt. % lymphocytes = 10%. WBC = 10,000.
$$\frac{10.0 \text{ X } 10,000}{100} = 1,000]$$

Early TLC: *1800 (normal) Refer to page 483*
Mid-hospitalization TLC: *1245 (mild deficiency)*
Most current TLC: *806 (Moderate deficiency, very close to severe which is measured as <800)*

      b.   What do the above trends tell you about this patient's immunocompetence status?
      It indicates that he is developing impaired immunocompetence which significantly increases his risk for developing infection.

E.   Physical Assessment for Protein and Protein-Calorie Malnutrition:

   1. Examine C.R.'s assessment data complete the following chart:

System	Presence (Yes/No)
1. Integumentary:	
-Decreased subcutaneous fat:	*Yes*
-Flaky, dry skin:	*Yes*
-Shedding of hair:	*No data*
2. Musculoskeletal:	
-Muscle wasting:	*Yes*
-Edema present:	*Yes*
3. Cardiovascular:	
-Evidence of decreased cardiac output:	*No data*
4. Evidence of lack of healing:	*Yes*

F. What conclusions can you draw from the preceding nutritional data?
   Mr. Cramer is suffering from both marasmus and kwashiokor types of malnutrition.

G. What factors have contributed to his current nutritional status?
   Hypermetabolic state, late initiation of nutritional support, possible inadequate nutritional support for his hypermetolic state.

H. Based on C.R.'s situation, what are the implications of waiting for a week or more before initiating nutritional support on this patient's status and prognosis?
   Starvation has a negative effect on the nutritional state of the patient. Catabolic processes have created a pattern of increasingly severe protein and protein-calorie malnutrition. It will be difficult to correct it.

I. What nursing diagnoses would you apply to C.R.'s plan of care based on this nutritional status?
   Alteration in nutrition: less than body requirement
   High risk for infection
   High risk for decreased cardiac output

J. What will be the focus of nursing management for C.R. related to his nutritional needs?
   Monitoring for therapeutic and possible nontherapeutic effects of his tube feedings. Accurate serial weight measurements. Close monitoring of his intake and output balance. Decreasing metabolic demands while maximizing nutritional supply.

[This patient was fortunate and did survive his tetanus episode. He remained in the ICU for approximately 4 months before he was able to resolve his multisystem dysfunctions. He returned to the unit approximately 6 months later to thank the nurses for his care.]

Case Study
The Case of Bob White

Mr. Bob White, a 60 year old retired business man, is brought into the emergency department in acute distress. His wife give a five day history of increasing symptoms of: shortness of breath, chest pain, ankle edema, and paroxysmal nocturnal dyspnea (PND). Mr. White finally allowed his wife to bring him in at 0200 because of a severe episode of PND associated with diaphoresis and unceasing chest pain.

Admission data included:

Vital Signs: BP = 160/94, HR = 110/minute, RR = 34/minute, Temp = 99 F
Chest Auscultation: Loud crackles up to midchest level, bilaterally
ECG: ST elevation and Q waves in V leads
Labs:

ABG: pH = 7.47, $PaCO_2$ = 28, PaO_2 = 55, SaO_2 = 86, HCO_3 = 20
Na = 137, K = 4.8, Cl = 97, Co_2 = 20, Glucose = 304, Creatinine = 1.2, BUN = 15

Cardiac Monitor: Showed sinus tachycardia with multifocal PVCs with some R on T phenomenon noted.

QUESTION: What does this cluster of data tell you about Mr. White's status?

DATA Continued:

Mr White now has a foley catheter inserted and his immediate urinary output is 65 cc of dark, concentrated urine. He is placed on 4 liters of nasal oxygen and taken to the coronary care unit. As the day progresses, Mr. White's condition progressively deteriorates. Hemodynamic monitoring devices are inserted and it is decided that he is now in cardiogenic shock. His cardiac enzyme levels are significantly elevated. His vital signs progressively worsen.

Suddenly, at 0500 on day two, Mr. White's cardiac monitor alarms. A run of ventricular tachycardia is noted, which rapidly degenerates into ventricular fibrillation. CPR is conducted and Mr. White is successfully treated after 45 minutes of CPR, now requiring large doses of drug support to maintain his blood pressure above a systolic of 90. IV lasix is repeatedly administered to maintain a urinary output of more than 25 cc/Hr.

24 hours following his cardiac arrest, lab values are now as follows:

Serum: Na = 130, K = 5.5, Creatinine = 5.4, Ca = 8.2, Albumin = 3.0
Urine: Na = 65, Osmolarity = 368, Creatinine = 5.2, +1 Protein
Urinary Output = 25-30 cc/Hr with drug support

72 hours followig his cardiac arrest, the following assessments are made:

He is very drowsy, opening his eyes for brief periods when stimulated. Skin coloring is pale and hot to the touch. His BP is now 174/95, HR = 125/minute. The cardiac monitor shows a sinus tachycardia with unifocal PVCs of less than 5/minute, at this time. His breathing is very deep and even, at 28/minute. Crackles are heard to mid-lung fields, bilaterally. Jugular vein distention is noted. He is unable to take in food orally. Bowel sounds are hyperactive and he had 5 liquid stools thus far this shift. His temperature is currently ranging from 100 - 102 F. His chest x-ray is positive for RUL pneumonia. He has just been placed on Gentamycin for treatment of the pneumonia. Urinary output is 27 cc/hr with drug and fluid support.

Lab values are now as follows:

Serum: Na = 131, K = 6.0, Creatinine = 3.8, BUN = 80, BUN/Creatinine ratio = 21, Ca = 7.8, Albumin = 2.5, CBC: RBC = 4.0, Hg = 11.5, Hct = 40, Platelets = 125,000

The Case of Bob White Study Guide

1. Admitting Diagnosis:

2. Relevant past medical and/or surgical history:

3. Recent History (Events leading to admission):

4. Focused Renal Dysfunction Assessment

   A. Did Mr. White experience any of the common causes of acute renal failure? (circle the number of the correct possible cause(s)

      1) Recent use of nephrotoxic substances

      2) Recent exposure to heavy metals or organic solvents

      3) Recent hypotensive episode of > 30 minutes

      4) Presence of tumor or multiple clots that might cause renovascular or urine outflow

         obstruction, bilaterally

   B. Physical Assessment Findings
      Examine the available physical assessment findings on Mr. White. Does he exhibit any of the following clinical findings of uremia? (place a check mark next to the body system that fits Mr. White's physical assessment)

Affected Body System	Common ARF Findings
_____ Neurologic	Decreased responsiveness level, drowsiness → coma; muscular twitching, and/or seizures?
_____ Cardiovascular	S/S of fluid volume excess? Cardiac arrhythmias? Metabolic acidosis? Electrolyte imbalances? Hypertension?
_____ Respiratory	S/S of recent pulmonary edema (fluid volume excess)? Kussmaul type respiratory pattern; Problems with airway clearance?
_____ Gastrointestinal	NG draining or feces positive for occult blood? anorexia? nausea &/or vomiting? constipation or diarrhea?
_____ Genitourinary	Urine output of < 25 to 30 mL/hr, even after fluid and/or diuretic management?
_____ Integumentary	Itchy and/or dry skin? Pale mucous membranes, coloring? Bruising present? Uremic frost present?
_____ Hematopoietic	RBC count < normal? Hgb & Hct < normal? Platelet count < normal? Any S/S of infection?
_____ General	General weakinss, fatigue? Activity intolerance? Metabolic Acidosis present?

QUESTION: Does Mr. White's laboratory data consistent with acute renal failure? (compare the A.R.F. data with Mr. White's data)

LABORATORY TEST	NORMAL VALUES	A.R.F. ABNORMAL TREND	TREND PRESENT (Yes / No))
SERUM:			
BUN	5-25 mg/dL	Increased	
Creatinine	0.5-1.5 mg/dL	Increased	
BUN/Creatinine Ratio	6-20 (mean = 10)	Increased	
Uric Acid	male: 3.5-8.0 mg/dL	Increased	
Potassium	3.5-5.3 mEq/L	Increased	
Calcium	9-11 mg/dL	Decreased	
Chloride	95-105 mEq/dL	Increased	
Phosphorus	2.5-4.5 mg/dL	Increased	
Albumin	3.5-5.0 g/dL	Decreased	
URINE:			
Protein	0-5 mg/dL/24 hr	Increased	
Creatinine Clearance	85-135 mL/min	Decreased	
Urea Clearance	64-100 mL/min	Decreased	

QUESTION: What do you notice about the relationship between serum and urine values of protein, creatinine and urea? What is happening?

QUESTION: Do Mr. White's actual laboratory trend indicate potential or actual acute renal failure?

7. Mr. White's data is most consistent with the risk of or presence of which type of acute renal failure? (Specify the most likely etiology)

Prerenal, caused by:

Intrarenal, caused by:

Postrenal, caused by:

QUESTION: If Mr. White has A.R.F. present, in which stage is he?

QUESTION: What would be your PRIORITY nursing diagnoses?

QUESTION: What would be the expected patient outcomes for this patient?

List 5 collaborative interventions that you would anticipate based on your nursing diagnoses.
1)

2)

3)

4)

5)

List 5 independent nursing interventions that you would anticipate, based on your nursing diagnoses:

1)

2)

3)

4)

5)

The Case of Bob White Study Guide
Instructor Guide

1. Admitting Diagnosis:
   Myocardial infarction and congestive heart failure

2. Relevant past medical and/or surgical history:
   Previous history unknown

3. Recent History (Events leading to admission):
   5 day history of increasing shortness of breath, edema and recurrent episodes of PND. Immediately prior to admission, experienced diaphoresis and unceasing chest pain

4. Focused Renal Dysfunction Assessment
   A. Did Mr. White experience any of the common causes of acute renal failure? (circle the number of the correct possible cause(s))
      1) Recent use of nephrotoxic substances – It is a concern that he was placed on Gentamycin which is nephrotoxic – he went into failure prior to
      2) Recent exposure to heavy metals or organic solvents
      3) Recent hypotensive episode of > 30 minutes: *Recent hypotensive episode of more than 30 minutes*
      4) Presence of tumor or multiple clots that might cause renovascular or urine outflow obstruction, bilaterally

   B. Physical Assessment Findings
      Examine the available physical assessment findings on Mr. White. Does he exhibit any of the following clinical findings of uremia? (place a check mark next to the body system that fits Mr. White's physical assessment)

Affected Body System	*Common ARF Findings*
__X__ Neurologic	*Decreased responsiveness level, drowsiness → coma; muscular twitching, and/or seizures?*
__X__ Cardiovascular	*S/S of fluid volume excess? Cardiac arrhythmias? Metabolic acidosis? Electrolyte imbalances? Hypertension?*
__X__ Respiratory	*S/S of recent pulmonary edema (fluid volume excess)? Kussmaul type respiratory pattern; Problems with airway clearance?*
__X__ Gastrointestinal	*NG draining or feces positive for occult blood? anorexia? nausea &/or vomiting? constipation or diarrhea?*
__X__ Genitourinary	*Urine output of < 25 to 30 mL/hr, even after fluid and/or diuretic management?*
__X__ Integumentary	*Itchy and/or dry skin? Pale mucous membranes, coloring? Bruising present? Uremic frost present?*
__X__ Hematopoietic	*RBC count < normal? Hgb & Hct < normal? Platelet count < normal? Any S/S of infection*
__X__ General	*General weakness, fatigue? Activity intolerance? Metabolic Acidosis present?*

QUESTION: Does Mr. White's laboratory data consistent with acute renal failure? (compare the A.R.F. data with Mr. White's data)

LABORATORY TEST	NORMAL VALUES	A.R.F. ABNORMAL TREND	TREND PRESENT (Yes / No))
SERUM:			
BUN	5-25 mg/dL	Increased	*Yes (70)*
Creatinine	0.5-1.5 mg/dL	Increased	*Yes (6.2)*
BUN/Creatinine Ratio	6-20 (mean = 10)	Increased	*Yes (21)*
Uric Acid	male: 3.5-8.0 mg/dL	Increased	*No data*
Potassium	3.5-5.3 mEq/L	Increased	*Yes (6)*
Calcium	9-11 mg/dL	*Decreased*	*Yes (7.8)*
Chloride	95-105 mEq/dL	Increased	*No data*
Phosphorus	2.5-4.5 mg/dL	Increased	*No data*
Albumin	3.5-5.0 g/dL	*Decreased*	*Yes (2.5)*
URINE:			
Protein	0-5 mg/dL/24 hr	Increased	*Yes*
Creatinine Clearance	85-135 mL/min	*Decreased*	*Yes (5.2)*
Urea Clearance	64-100 mL/min	*Decreased*	*No data*

QUESTION: What do you notice about the relationship between serum and urine values of protein, creatinine and urea? What is happening? *They maintain an inverse relationship – as serum levels decrease (or increase) the urine levels shift in the opposite direction. When the kidneys do not filter, serum levels increase, thus decreasing the amount the moves into the urine to be excreted. Protein, however, leaks out of the kidneys, into the urine.*

QUESTION: Do Mr. White's actual laboratory trends indicate potential or actual acute renal failure? *Yes*

7. Mr. White's data is most consistent with the risk of or presence of which type of acute renal failure? (Specify the most likely etiology)

       Prerenal, caused by: *Prolonged hypotensive episode secondary to cardiac failure & cardiac arrest.*
       Intrarenal, caused by:
       Postrenal, caused by:

QUESTION: If Mr. White has A.R.F. present, in which stage is he? *Onset Stage – His urine output has not dropped sufficiently to be considered as oliguric/anuric*

QUESTION: What would be your PRIORITY nursing diagnoses?
       Fluid volume excess
       High risk for injury r/t electrolyte imbalance
       Decreased cardiac output
       Infection

QUESTION: What would be the management goals for Mr White?
       Appropriate goals include:
           Treat the underlying cause
               Need to increase cardiac output to increase tissue perfusion. he is at risk for developing acute tubular necrosis. Further hypotensive episodes will damage his already dysfunctional kidney's even further.
       Maintain normal normal fluid volume
               He will likely require dialysis to remove excess fluid until his kidneys can excrete sufficient quantities. He may also be maintained on a tight fluid restriction

Prevent complications
> *Because acute renal failure can lead to multisystem dysfunction, it will be important to monitor him closely for complications such as infection, extension of his MI, metabolic acidosis, and other problems.*

List 5 collaborative interventions that you would anticipate based on your nursing diagnoses.
1) *Dialysis*

2) *Laboratory tests: electrolytes, BUN, creatinine, uric acid, ABG, etc.*

3) *Chest x-rays*

4) *IV fluid orders*

5) *Drug therapy: Antibiotics (note that he just had Gentamycin ordered). Cardiac drug therapy*

List 5 independent nursing interventions that you would anticipate, based on your nursing diagnoses:
1) *Daily weights – monitor I:O strictly*

2) *Strict intake control and documentation*

3) *Monitor closely for clinical manifestations of fluid volume excess*

4) *Turn every 2 hours*

5) *Frequent vital sign checks*

6) *Cardiac monitoring – monitor for increase in dysrhythmias*

PROBLEM SOLVING EXERCISES
Suggestions For Use

Problem Solving Exercises take about 1 to 1 ½ hours to complete, depending on the length of time students are given to discuss things in their small groups.

1. Do not inform students about the outcome focus. The object of the exercise is to assist in learning clinical problem solving. The first half of the exercise involves developing nursing hypotheses which require knowledge of disease processes. The second half of the exercise involves developing a plan of care based on available data base.

2. If possible, break students into groups of approximately 7-10. If not possible, the exercise can be done as a large group effort. Ideally, there are a variety of supportive texts available in the room (lab manuals, drug manuals, med/surg texts).

3. The instructor becomes the patient and presents the scenario, answering questions each group asks.

4. Each group is asked to decide (and agree) on 4 major patient problems based on the preliminary data.

5. Each group is given a sheet of paper to write down questions they wish to ask the patient. Students are told the questions should relate to data collection (e.g. history, physical exam, labs, etc.).

6. Begin the first round of questions. Each group is allowed to ask one question. They are told to ask what they consider to be the highest priority assessment question. Instructor answers, solely based on the instructor's data sheet. Instructor can indicate in provided space, when each bit of data is requested. If students ask for data not included in the provided data base - state "no data is available". Do not volunteer data. (It is a good idea to make notations of questions that students ask that are not present in the instructor data sheet – they can be examined later for possible incorporation into the scenario for its next use.)

7. Let students discuss for brief time (about 5 minutes), the data they obtained from the first round of questions. Begin second round of questions, based on the data obtained in the first round. Each group is allowed one question. Again, ask for what they believe is the most important data to obtain.

8. Let students discuss new data base for brief time (5 minutes). Begin third (final) round of questions. Each group is able to ask two questions.

9. Students are then instructed to cluster their data, based on all of the data they have asked for. They can also be requested to write down any further data they wish they could obtain to help confirm their hypothesis.

10. The remainder of the exercise (nursing process) can either be done during the first 30 minutes of the next class period or could be done as a take home exercise. Either way, students are to use available resources to develop a plan of care based on their data base.

Problem Solving Exercise
The Case of C.R. Cramer
A Patient With a Complex Health Problem

On the third of March of this year Mr. C.R. Cramer, a 50 year old store owner, stepped on a nail while carrying boxes in his store. Rather than seeking medical attention, he cleaned the wound on his left foot and continued to work. On the 4th post injury day, C.R. noted slight weakness and stiffness in his legs and a tightening of his jaw. By day #6, he asked to be taken to the local emergency department. At that time, his joints were very stiff and he could no longer open his mouth. Upon being diagnosed with tetanus, C.R. was rapidly transferred to this regional medical center in mild respiratory distress which rapidly deteriorated, requiring mechanical ventilation. In the ICU, he is placed on neuromuscular blockade IV drug therapy to paralyze him. C.R. received a right below the knee amputation on day as a result of an uncontrolled infection.

C.R. has now been in the hospital for 8 days. The nursing staff is concerned about his increasing generalized edema and fever. His general condition remains unstable.

Task #1

Based only on the available data, develop a list of at least four possible etiologies of C.R.'s edema.

1.

2.

3.

4.

5.

Task #2

Using a clean sheet of paper, write down: 1) questions you would like to ask C.R.'s nurse or physician. 2) assessments you would perform, and/or 3) tests that you would like to see obtained in developing an hypothesis.

[At this point, the spokesperson in each group is given the opportunity to ask one question to develop a specific data base]

Task #3

Examine all of the available data up to this point. Cluster the data beginning with the most critical cues, into relevant conceptual patterns problems. If available, use your reference books to help you understand the significance of the data that you may be unfamiliar with.

CLUSTER #1:

CLUSTER #2:

CLUSTER #3:

CLUSTER #4:

Task #4

Based on the data you have now available, what do you believe are C.R.'s acute health problems?

PART TWO OF CASE

Task #5

Based on the existing data, the team tentatively concludes that C.R. is experiencing a state of hypercatabolism, hypermetabolism and malnutrition. He is also immunocompromised. What other information could the nurse or physician collect that will confirm or refute this diagnosis? Identify at least 3 items.

1.

2.

3.

4.

Task #6

Why was C.R. at risk for a nutritional/immune deficiency? Work with your group and list 3 reasons. Explain the relationship between the item and nutritional/immune status.

Potential reasons for nutrition/immune problems	Nutritional Relationship
1.	
2.	
3.	
4.	
5.	

Task #7

List appropriate nursing diagnoses that apply to C.R.'s nutritional/immune deficits and number them according to priority.

FACULTY GUIDE: HISTORY / ASSESSMENT DATA
The Case of C.R. Cramer

PARAMETER / TEST	Requested Data	DATA
Serial weights		Admission: 205, Day #2 210, Day #4 203, current: 182
Cardiovascular		S1 and S2. 3+ generalized edema is noted.
Neurological		Remains on Norcuron drip -- paralyzed.
Diet		Not receiving any nutritional supplement as yet.
Bowel function		Diarrhea. Rectal bag is in place.
BKA wound flap site		Several open lesions are noted with white patches. Has continuing drainage.
Skin / mucous membranes		Skin is dray and shedding. His flesh is beginning to hang. A small decubitus is noted on his coccyx. His oral mucous membranes have white patches.
Medical History		5 year history of non-insulin dependent D.M. - usually diet controlled. Has a history of MI, one year ago and one episode of CHF. Has arthritis.
Allergies		Penicillin
Smoking / ETOH history		Has smoked 1 PPD for 22 years. No use of alcohol.
Height		6 Foot, 1 inch, large framed
Lung sounds		Rhonchi throughout lungs.
Chest X-ray		RLL pneumonia. Notes a RLL fluid mass that may be empyema.
Mid-arm Circumference		Admission: 28.4 cm Current: 27.3 cm
WBC & Lymphs		Admission: WBC = 18,200, Lymphs = 9.9% Most current: 12,400, Lymphs = 6.5% Other: current Bands = 10%
Serum Albumin Prealbumin Protein		Adm.: 3.5 mg/dL Prealbumin = 18 Current: 1.8 mg/dL Total protein level: 5.8 (nl = 6.6-7.9)
Nitrogen Balance Measurement		24 hour Ntg intake: 54.3 g/24 hrs. (nl = 56/24 hrs.) 24 hour Ntg excretion: 62.1g/24 hrs.
Dietary history		Cousins report: Lives alone. Us usually a good eater but does not watch what he eats very well to control his DM. His appetite decreased steadily because he felt so "poorly" following foot injury.

PARAMETER / TEST	Requested Data	DATA
Urine status		A foley catheter is in place. His urine output has been consistently > 30 mL/Hr. Urine appears yellow and slightly cloudy.
IV fluids		5% Dextrose and NS with 20 KCL at 100 mL/Hr.
Medications		Heparin drip : 1,000 units per hour Versed Drip at 8 mg/hr Insulin per sliding scale Nystatin swish/spit Nystatin powder to stump q 6 hrs. IV antibiotics
EKG		Sinus tachycardia. Appearance is consistent with MI of undetermined age.
Wound Culture of flap		Shows candida albicans.
ABG results		pH - 7.44; PCO_2 - 35, PO_2 - 92, HCO_3 - 24 Pulse oximetry: 92 %
Temperature		Axillary: 100.4
BP and P		104/68, P 116, regular; Pulse characteristic = normal
Abdomen		Distended.
Electrolytes		K = 3.2, Phosphate = 2.0 (nl = 2.4-4.7 mg/dL, Mg = 1.4 (nl 1.8-3 mg/dL) Na = 126, Ca = 4.3 mEq/L.
BUN & Creatinine		BUN = 45, Creatinine = 1.0
Blood Glucose		200

Clinical Focus: Endocrine Problem (Diabetes Mellitus)

Student Name: _____. Date: _____

Patient Initials: _____. Age: _____. Gender: _____. Adm. Date: _____.

Admission Dx.: _____

_____

==

ASSESSMENT

1. Documented endocrine disease or risk factors present for development of (e.g., obesity):

2. Physical Examination:

   Assess for the following chronic complications in a patient with diabetes mellitus (DM):

Complication	Clinical symptoms	If present, describe:
Peripheral neuropathies	pain, abnormal sensations, local anesthesia	
Macrovascular disease	decreased arterial blood flow (gangrene, pain, loss of peripheral pulses, angina)	
Retinopathy	blindness, small vessel hemorrhage(s) in retina	
Nephropathy	elevated serum creatinine, BUN levels, decreased U/O	
Infection	fever, elevated WBCs, pain	
Poor wound healing	slough (moist, stringy, thick yellow tissue that is dying), eschar (black, hard, necrotic tissue), poor wound closure	

4. What psychologic or physiologic stressors is your patient currently experiencing?

5. Infection is the main trigger for both DKA and HHNK in the diabetic patient. Identify the presence of clinical indicators of infection in your patient.

    - Elevated WBC count: () yes () no
    - Fever   () yes () no
    - Cloudy urine   () yes () no
    - Green/yellow sputum   () yes () no
    - Adventitious breath sounds   () yes () no
    - Purulent drainage   () yes () no
    - Positive cultures   () yes () no – if positive, identify source:

6. The following laboratory studies are important to assess in patients with DM. Document & analyze the most current values on your patient. Explain variations and treatment.

Test	Patient's Test Result	Elevated, decreased, normal?	Treatment given, if any
SERUM			
• Glucose			
• Potassium			
• Sodium			
• Ketone			
• pH			
• Phosphorus			
URINE			
• Glucose			
• Ketones			

ANALYSIS

7. Based on the data you have collected, is this patient at risk for developing any of the following: DKA, HHNK, or hypoglycemia?   Explain why or why not.

PLANNING

8. Based on your analysis, what interventions can you plan to prevent this patient from developing a diabetic crisis?

9. Planning insulin management. Complete the following section to enhance your knowledge about insulin administration.

Regular Insulin
Action:

Appearance: Type of syringe used to administer:

Dosage increments: Route of administration:

Time of action onset: Time drug peaks:

When would signs of hypoglycemia most likely occur?

What interventions would you do to treat hypoglycemia on this patient?

NPH Insulin
Action:

Appearance: Type of syringe used to administer:

Dosage increments: Route of administration:

Time of action onset: Time drug peaks:

When would signs of hypoglycemia most likely occur?

What interventions would you do to treat hypoglycemia on this patient?

10. What type of teaching does this patient need prior to discharge? Develop a teaching plan to treat a knowledge deficit regarding one of the broad topics.

Broad Topics
Insulin administration; signs and treatment of hypoglycemia & hyperglycemia; foot & skin care; glucose monitoring; diabetic diet; prevention of chronic complications

Broad Topic: _____

Learning Objectives	How Patient/Family Will Demonstrate Comptence

CLINICAL FOCUS: ACUTE GI PROBLEMS

Student Name: _____ Date: _____

Patient Initials: _____. Admission Date: _____. Age: _____. Gender: _____.

Admitting Diagnosis: _____

_____

Circumstances surrounding admission: _____

_____.

Past Medical History / Surgeries &/or Major Procedures: _____

_____

****

ASSESSMENT

1. Patient History
    A. Risk factors
        Pre-existing (exposure to toxins; alcohol/drug use; biliary tract disease (gallstones); recent trauma; environment and/or occupational)

        Hospitalization related factors (drugs; hypotensive episodes, etc.):

2. Physical Assessment
    Assess your patient for the following complications.

	Clinical Symptoms	If Present in Patient, describe:
Comfort	• Abdominal pain (include location, severity, precipitating factors, relief measures); • Pruritis	
Nutrition	• Nausea & vomiting &/or diarrhea (include association with food or alcohol intake). • Recent food & liquid intake (include any food intolerances). • Abdominal distention	
Fluid & Electrolyte	• Weight loss or gain (past 6 months) • S/S fluid/electrolyte deficit (weakness, dizziness, syncope, tetany, poor skin turgor, dry lips & mucous membranes) • S/S fluid & electrolyte excess (edema in hands, feet, legs; increase in abdominal girth)	
Neurologic	• S/S of encephalopathy; hand &/or feet tremor	

	Clinical Symptoms	If Present in Patient, describe:
Cardiovascular	• Blood pressure (including orthostatic changes), pulse, temperature elevation	
Respiratory	• Respiratory rate/pattern, and breath sounds	
Abdomen	• Tenderness or rigidity • Presence of bowel sounds (including quality, location • Presence of Grey Turner's sign &/or Cullen's sign • Presence of abdominal distention, ascites (tight, glistening skin with bulging flanks & presence of fluid wave & shifting dullness on percussion)	
Integumentary	• Jaundice (most integumentary findings fall in other categories)	
Elimination	• Clay colored stools/dark or bloody urine; + guaiac stools	
General	• Affect, mental status, responsiveness (note facial expression	

Laboratory Assessment

Assess your patient's most current lab values

Serum Laboratory Test -- normal values	This Patient's Values	Abnormal Trend (↑,↓)	Interpretation
Glucose –			
Potassium –			
Calcium –			
Chloride –			
Phosphate –			
BUN –			

Serum Laboratory Test -- normal values	This Patient's Values	Abnormal Trend ($\uparrow,\downarrow$)	Interpretation
Creatinine –			
Amylase –			
Lipase –			
Albumin –			
AST –			
ALT –			
GGT –			
Alk. Phosphatase –			
Ammonia –			
PTT –			
PT –			

ANALYSIS

QUESTION: Do this patient's actual lab trends and physical assessment indicate possible or actual pancreatitis and/or liver dysfunction?   If "yes", explain your answer.

Based on the data you have collected, what would be your priority nursing diagnosis?

PLANNING

List 5 collaborative interventions that you would anticipate based on your nursing diagnosis.

List 5 independent nursing interventions that you would anticipate, based on your nursing diagnosis.

What type of teaching or other activities need to be conducted with the patient and/or family in anticipation of transfer or discharge?

PART VII

INJURY

PART VII. INJURY

Take Home Cases (THC)
       Complex Wound Management (Module 28)   273
       Acute Burn Injury (Module 29)   275

Case Studies
       The Case of Mary Mole   278
       The Case of Bobby W.   282

Problem Solving Exercise (PSE)
       The Case of Mike Brady   293

Clinical Focus: Injury   299

Take Home Case
Module 28: Complex Wound Management

Student name:_____   Date:_____

Directions
        Using the appropriate reading assignments complete the following questions or statements using complete sentences.

****

Section one:
1. The main role of the subcutaneous tissue is to _____.

Section two:
2. List the methods of wound closure appropriate for primary intention:

Section three:
3. How do steroids interfere with wound healing?

Section four:
4. What is the most important act to prevent wound infections?

Section five:
5. The purpose of wet to dry dressings is:

6. Polyurethane films are used to dress draining or infected wounds.

        True or False (circle one)

Section six:
7. List methods for determining local perfusion of a wound.

Section seven:
8. Describe a stage II pressure ulcer.

Section eight:
9. How often should a pressure ulcer be reassessed to examine healing?

        10. How should pressure ulcers be managed?

Take Home Case
Module 28: Complex Wound Management
Instructor Guide

1. Regulate body temperature
   Provide the body with shape and substance.

2. sutures
   staples
   steri-strips/tape

3. Decreases protein synthesis
   Delays development of granulation tissue
   Inhibits fibroblasts
   Reduces epithelialization

4. Handwashing

5. To remove debris and provide a moist wound environment

6. False

7. Presence of debris indicates decreased perfusion ability
   Skin temperature
   Capillary refill
   Presence of proximal and distal pulses around the wound

8. Partial thickness skin loss. Superficial abrasion, blister or shallow crater.

9. Once a week.

10. Proper positioning to raise pressure ulcer off the bed
    Debridement, cleansing, dressing changes
    Proper support surface for patient

Take Home Case
Module 29: Acute Burn Injury

Student name:_____   Date:_____

DIRECTIONS:
    Using the appropriate reading assignment, complete the following questions or statements using complete sentences.
****

Situation: M.J. is a 45 year old male who has sustained a 60% full thickness burn to his chest, face, arms, and thighs after falling asleep on the sofa while smoking. Upon admission to the ED, he is noted to be alert, crying out in pain and to have stridor.

Section two:
1.   Describe the appearance of M.J.'s full thickness burn:_____

Section four:
2.   M.J.'s stridor is an indication he has suffered an _____ injury.
        A.   List 3 other signs of this injury:

                _____

                _____

                _____

        B.   List labs that support the diagnosis of this condition:

3.   In the first 24 hours post burn injury. M.J.'s hypovolemic shock is caused by:_____

_____

Please describe the pathophysiology of this phenomena:

_____

_____

4.   M.J. weighs 100 Kg. Calculate his fluid resuscitation needs during his 3rd post-burn hour using the Parkland Formula.

_____

_____

Section five:
5.   During the emergent period, the preferred drug/route of choice for M.J.'s pain control is intramuscular morphine.
        True or False (circle one)

Section seven:
6.   The acute phase of burn care begins at _____ and

    ends when _____.

Section eight:

7. The two major nursing actions aimed at the prevention of wound infections are:

    a._____

    b._____

8. Superficial partial thickness wounds heal by _____.

9. Give an example of a temporary biologic dressing that might be used in M.J.'s care:

Section nine:

10. A _____ diet will be necessary to meet M.J.'s nutritional demands secondary to his hypermetabolism.

Section eleven:

11. Functional deficits occur over joints due to what normal mechanism of wound healing?

Take Home Case:
Module 29: Acute Burn Injury
Instructor Guide

1. Skin is leathery in texture. Wound is white or charred.

2. Inhalation injury
    a. facial burns
       cough
       wheezes
       tachypnea
       singed nasal hair
       enclosed space burn
       flash burn
    b. abnormal ABGs
       elevated carboxyhemoglobin levels

3. Vasodilation and increased capillary permeability
Loss of capillary seal leading to fluid and electrolyte shifts from intravascular to initial spaces

4. 4 ml LR x 60% x 100 Kg = total amount to be infused
    divided by 2 = total amount to be infused first 8 hours post injury
    divided by 8 = hourly infusion amount

5. False
intravenous morphine

6. 48 to 72 hours post injury
all wounds are healed

7. irrigation and debridement
protective isolation
applying topical antibiotics
sterile application of dressings

8. Spontaneous reepithelialization

9. homograft (human cadaver)
heterograft (non human/animal)

10. high calorie, high protein

11. Excessive edema impairs ROM and results in fibrosis and contractures. Edema is a normal response to wound healing.

Case Study
The Case of Mary Mole
A Patient with a Wound Management Problem

SITUATION:

Mary Mole is admitted to your unit following a motor vehicle crash. She is admitted for observation since she has hematuria and she is one year status post renal transplant. She sustained multiple facial lacerations. You are asked to assist the plastic surgeon as she repairs the lacerations.

QUESTION #1: Which method of wound closure do you anticipate will be used?

****

While talking with Mrs. Mole you discover she is an insulin controlled diabetic. She laughs and states, "that is the least of my worries, I'm 50 pounds overweight!" Current medications include: Lasix (10 mg QD), Folic acid (QD), 5 units regular and 10 units NPH insulin Q am, 15 units NPH insulin Q pm, Solu-medrol (5 mg QD), Imuran (400 mg QD).

****

QUESTION #2: Which factors in Mrs. Mole's history places her at risk for wound healing and why?

QUESTION #3: The physician repairs the lacerations and asks you to dress the wounds. What type of dressing would best promote healing?

****

Mrs. Mole complains of abdominal pain as the shift progresses. Her abdomen becomes firm and tender on palpation. Bowel sounds disappear. The decision is made to take her for an exploratory laparotomy. An intestinal tear is discovered and repaired. She returns to your unit post-op. She has an abdominal dressing in place with a sump drain.

****

QUESTION #4: What equipment will the nurse need in order to operate the sump drain?

QUESTION #5: The physician writes an order for a wet-to-damp dressing using saline. Why?

QUESTION #6: Which of the following is true about a wet-to-damp dressing? (check one)

a) it must be changed frequently

b) solution should be dripping from the dressing

c) the wound should be tightly packed

d) gauze touching the wound should be folded

[This ends the case of Mary Mole]

Case Study
The Case of Mary Mole
A Patient with a Wound Management Problem
Instructor's Guide
[The following case study can be used if the instructor wishes to emphasize principles discussed in Module #28: Complex Wound Management]

Mary Mole is admitted to your unit following a motor vehicle crash. She is admitted for observation since she has hematuria and she is one year status post renal transplant. She sustained multiple facial lacerations. You are asked to assist the plastic surgeon as she repairs the lacerations.

QUESTION #1: Which method of wound closure do you anticipate will be used?

>   ANSWER: *Primary intention since these wounds are usually superficial with minimal tissue loss. Secondary intention would produce greater scarring.*

****

While talking with Mrs. Mole you discover she is an insulin controlled diabetic. She laughs and states, "that is the least of my worries, I'm 50 pounds overweight!" Current medications include: Lasix (10 mg QD), Folic acid (QD), 5 units regular and 10 units NPH insulin Q am, 15 units NPH insulin Q pm, Solu-medrol (5 mg QD), Imuran (400 mg QD).

****

QUESTION #2: Which factors in Mrs. Mole's history places her at risk for wound healing and why?

>   ANSWER:
>   *Diabetes:*   *Small vessel vascular changes impair tissue perfusion.*
>   *Obesity:*   *Fatty tissue is poorly vascularized, although this may not be a problem with facial wounds, her obesity may reflect malnutrition and protein deficit*
>   *Folic acid:*   *Is she anemic? If so, decreased oxygen delivery to wounds*
>   *Solu-Medrol:*   *Inhibits inflammatory response, delays development of granulation tissue*
>   *Imuran:*   *Predisposes the wounds to infection secondary to immunosuppression, decreases T and B lymphocyte production*

QUESTION #3: The physician repairs the lacerations and asks you to dress the wounds. What type of dressing would best promote healing?

>   ANSWER: *Dry dressing*

****

Mrs. Mole complains of abdominal pain as the shift progresses. Her abdomen becomes firm and tender on palpation. Bowel sounds disappear. The decision is made to take her for an exploratory laparotomy. An intestinal tear is discovered and repaired. She returns to your unit post-op. She has an abdominal dressing in place with a sump drain.

****

QUESTION #4: What equipment will the nurse need in order to operate the sump drain?

>   ANSWER: *A wall suction system.*

QUESTION #5: The physician writes an order for a wet to damp dressing using Hydrogen peroxide and saline. Why?

ANSWER: *It will aid mechanical debridement and not damage granulation tissue.*

QUESTION #6: Which of the following is true about a wet to damp dressing?
a) it must be changed frequently
b) solution should be dripping from the dressing
c) the wound should be tightly packed
d) gauze touching the wound should be folded

ANSWER: *a) It must be changed frequently*

[This ends the case of Mary Mole]

Case Study
The Case of Bobby W.
A Complex Patient with Nutrition and Immunocompetence Problems

PART I: BOBBY'S ADMISSION

Recent History

On February 3 of this year, Bobby W. was referred to your hospital from a small outlying hospital for treatment of a severe thermal injury. The referring hospital reports that Bobby was welding pipe in an oil field when the pipe broke. A mixture of gas and oil began leaking from the pipe and subsequently exploded. Bobby sustained a flash injury. He reportedly drove himself to the local hospital, walking into the Emergency Department alert and oriented. Intravenous fluids were initiated immediately. Shortly thereafter, Bobby began coughing up carbonaceous sputum and developed respiratory distress, requiring intubation. He was then transported by ambulance to your facility. The ambulance run took approximately 4 hours. He is diagnosed with a 60% BSA burn.

Past History

Bobby W. is 29 years of age. He is married with three small children. At the time of the event, he was working as a driller for Dillon Drilling Co. in Ashford, Kentucky. He is a heavy smoker, according to his wife, smoking 2 to 3 packs per day. Bobby has been in very good health prior to this admission. He has been on no medications at home. He has no known allergies and has no apparent chronic medical problems.

The Initial Appraisal

You are a nurse in the Burn Unit and you have been assigned to care for Bobby today. You have just walked into his cubical to perform a rapid initial appraisal.

General appearance: Your first impression of Bobby is that he is severely compromised at this time. His head, trunk and extremities are burned and his hair is singed off. He appears somewhat restless at this time. His eyes dart around the room and he makes grabbing motions with his right hand, as you approach the bed.

Signs of distress: He is lying on his back, restlessly moving his head and extremities.

Skin Color: You are unable to assess due to the extensiveness of his flash burns.

Responsiveness Level: Bobby moves his extremities with purpose and looks at you when you talk, but is uncooperative.

Presence of supportive or monitoring devices: Bobby has an oral endotracheal tube in place and is on the Bear-5 mechanical ventilator at:
Tidal Volume of 650 mL, FiO_2 of 50%, Assist/Control Mode at 12 breaths per minute.
He has a urinary catheter in place. He is attached to a cardiac monitor which shows a normal sinus rhythm.

Other: He has a triple lumen central venous line in place in the right subclavian. Lactated Ringers is currently infusing. A nasogastric tube is in place to low wall suction.
Bobby is 5' 11' tall and usually weighs 155 pounds.

Systemic Bedside Assessment

Head and Neck
Bobby has a Glasgow Coma Scale score of 10-T (Eye = 4, Motor = 5, Verbal = 1-T). He will not follow commands but moves all extremities with purpose. He has charring of his lower face and neck. His upper face and ears are also burned. His hair is severely singed. A 7.5 oral endotracheal tube is in place. His face is edematous with eyes swollen shut and reddened tongue.

Chest
Upper chest is burned and blistering is present.

Pulmonary status: Bilateral breath sounds are noted, with decreased sounds in the right upper lung field. He is breathing with the assistance of the mechanical ventilator. He is requiring suctioning approximately every hour for moderate amounts of gray/white secretions.

Cardiac status: He continues in a sinus tachycardia. S_1 and S_2 and a soft murmur are auscultated. His current blood pressure is 170/60, taken in his right thigh.

Abdomen

Abdomen is flat. Bowel sounds absent all 4 quads. The skin on lower abdomen is not burned.

Pelvis

He is uncircumcised. His anterior pelvic & genitalia area are not burned. urinary catheter in place. The urine is dark amber colored with a specific gravity of 1.030 and 2+ ketones.

Extremities:

Both hands and arms are burned (skin blistering and skin loss noted). Poor capillary refill in hands. No radial pulses are palpable. Pulses in feet are decreased.

Posterior:

buttocks and lower back burned and blistering but upper back spared. difficult to assess back well because his condition requires that he lie on his back or tilt only slightly to either side.

Vital Signs:

BP = 170/60; P = 135; regular; R = 24/minute, T = 99.7, rectally

Initial Labs

CBC: Hgb = 17.5, Hct = 49, WBC = 14,000, RBC = 5.4

ABG: pH = 7.54, PaO_2 = 80, $PaCO_2$ = 27, HCO_3 = 26

Selected Medical Team Findings and Progress Notes From admission to Current Time

1. Dietary Consult of 2/12:
    3,500 Cal/day (50 Cal/Kg) and > 100 Gm Protein/day needed.
    [2/17: A High Nutrition (HN) tube feeding was ordered to run initially at 25 cc/hr]
2. Note on 2/29: Wounds smell like pseudomonas.
3. Note on 3/6: Began first series of debridement and grafting. Also performed excision of burn eschar with split thickness skin graft (STSG) to both hands.
4. Note on 3/24: Labs show staphylococcus aureus on face and candida albicans on skin culture.
5. Note on 3/25: Temperature remains elevated. R/O sub-bacterial endocarditis. Remains confused.
6. Cardiology Consult:
    Murmur heard, more prominent than on admission. Spiking temperature. Various staph. growth on Swan-Ganz and CVP tips. Echocardiogram done - negative.
7. Note on 3/27: Blood cultures show staphylococcus aureus.
    ****

PART II: BOBBY, EIGHT WEEKS FOLLOWING ADMISSION

Most Current Status Report:

T = 100.4 (R); Intake = 3920 mL and Output = 1475 mL over the past 24 hours. Continues to have scattered open areas over burn fields. Scattered light rhonchi are present that clear somewhat with coughing. He has positive bowel sounds. A urinary catheter remains in place. Current weight is 138 pounds.

Current Medication Orders Included:

Multivits Liquid, Zinc Sulfate Cap., Ascorbic Acid Liqiod
Nafcillin Injection

Significant Labs (Abnormals only)

WBC : 12.0, Lymphocyte count = 9%, **Hg:** 11.3, **Hct** : 33.6

Electrolytes: Na = 128 mEq/L, Cl = 97 meq/L , K = 2.9 mEq/L, PO_4 = 1.8 mg/dL, Mg = 1.2 mEq/L, Total Calcium = 4.1 mg/dL.

Serum Albumin = 1.9 g/dL

24 hour Urine Urea Nitrogen = 15.4 g,   **Nitrogen Intake** = 21 g

Tube feeding information:

Ensure Plus tube feeding which supplies 55 g/L of protein and 1.5 Cal/mL. It is infusing at 100 cc/hr.

The Case of Bobby W.: Study Guide

1.   Significant Past Medical and Social History:

Are their any factors present in his history that might influence his nutritional status?

2.   Nutritional Assessment

    A.   Dietary History

        1.   Pre-existing nutritional status:

        2.   Length of time patient on NPO status (prior to initiation of P, intralipids, tube feedings):

        3.   Nutrition Orders (specify existing orders):

        Tube Feedings:
        Vitamin and/or mineral supplements:
        P.O. Diet:

    B.   Nitrogen Balance

        1.   Latest Urine Urea Nitrogen (UUN) results:

        2.   Is he in positive nitrogen balance?
        [Base your answer by using this chart data: The dietary consult states that Bobby's protein intake is _____/24 hour period.]

    C.   Weight Status

    Bobby weighed _____ pounds prior to admission. Currently he weighs _____ pounds. This represents a _____percent weight loss.

    Is this percent of weight loss significant? If yes, in what way?

    D.   Protein Measurement

        1.   Visceral Protein

            a.   Bobby's serum albumin is_____g/dL. What is the significance of this value to Bobby's nutritional status?

E. **Physical Assessment for Protein and Protein-Calorie Malnutrition:**

The following are typical clinical findings consistent with protein-calorie malnutrition. Which could be assessed in Bobby's situation? Does he have any of these present?

System	Able to Assess	Present (Yes/No)
Integumentary:		
-Decreased subu fat	_____	_____
-Flaky, dry skin	_____	_____
-Shedding of hair	_____	_____
Musculoskeletal:		
-Muscle wasting	_____	_____
-Edema present	_____	_____
Cardiovascular:		
-Evidence of dec. C.O.	_____	_____
Evidence of lack of healing:	_____	_____

F. **What conclusions can you draw from the nutritional data you have gathered here?**

G. **Examine Bobby's Serum Electrolytes:**

Electrolyte	Normal Range	Bobby's Value
Sodium	135 - 145 mEq/L	_____
Chloride	96 - 106 mEq/L	_____
Potassium	3.5 - 5.5 mEq/L	_____
Total Calcium	4.3 - 5.5 mEq/L	_____
Phosphorus	3.0 - 4.5 mg/dL	_____
Magnesium	1.5 - 2.2 mEq/L	_____

1. Why are they abnormal?

2. Which one(s) should be addressed FIRST? Why?

3. Does Bobby currently exhibit any clinical manifestations that are consistent with any of these electrolyte deficits?

H.   Is Bobby in a hypermetabolic state? If he is, when will it cease to exist?

I.   Immunocompetence Assessment

      A.   Which of the following critical cues suggesting immunocompetence problems does Bobby exhibit, if any?

Critical Cue	Present (Y/N)
Fever	_____
Poor wound healing	_____
Abnormal CBC with Diff.	_____
Abnormal coagulation studies	_____
Recurrent, prolonged, or severe infections	_____
Secondary infections	_____
Immunosuppressive drug therapy	_____
Other at-risk factors	_____

      B.   Total Lymphocyte Count (TLC)

           1.   Examine the most recent CBC with diff. Using the given formula, determine the TLC.

$$TLC = \frac{\%\ Lymphocytes \times WBC}{100}$$

[Exa. Pt % lymphs = 10%, WBC =10,000:]

$$TLC = \frac{10.0 \times 10,000}{100} = 1,000$$

           2.   Bobby's TLC is currently _____.

      C.   What do the available data tell you about Bobby's immunocompetence status?

      D.   What is the relationship between Bobby's malnutrition status and his immunocompetence status?

3.   Nursing Implications

    A.   List 5 nursing diagnoses that would be appropriate based on this data base:

      1.

      2.

      3.

      4.

      5.

B.   What would be the major expected patient outcomes for Bobby based on the nursing diagnoses you have developed?

C.   List 5 collaborative interventions that you would anticipate based on your nursing diagnoses:

D.   List 5 independent nursing interventions that your would anticipate, based on your nursing diagnoses:

Case Study
The Case of Bobby W. Study Guide
Instructor Guide

Note: The Case of Bobby W. is a reality based case presentation. The data available may show evidence of multiple problem areas. You may focus on burn care and principles outlined in Module 29 by developing questions to focus on grafting and infection. The focus taken in the instruction manual is on nutrition and can be used in conjunction with Module 20. Thus, most of the questions in this exercise will center around consideration of his nutrition/immunocompetence status.

1.   **Significant Past Medical and Social History:**
      Heavy smoker; On no medications at home; In good health; No known allergies

      Are their any factors present in his history that might influence his nutritional status?
      It is to his advantage that he was in good health prior to admission. His normal weight was within the 50th percentile for his age and height (medium frame).

2.   **Nutritional Assessment**

      A.   **Dietary History**
            1.   Pre-existing nutritional status: *Good*
            2.   Length of time patient on NPO status (prior to initiation of TPN, intralipids, tube feedings): *According to available chart data it looks like he was started on tube feedings on day 14. There is no record of having received prior nutritional support.*

            3.   Nutrition Orders (specify existing orders):

                  Tube Feedings: *Ensure Plus tube feeding which supplies 55 g/L of protein and 1.5 Cal/mL. It is infusing at 100 cc/hr.*
                  Vitamin and/or mineral supplements: *Yes, refer to medication list*
                  P.O. Diet: *None indicated*

      B.   **Nitrogen Balance**
            1.   Latest Urine Urea Nitrogen (UUN) results: *15.4 g/24 hours*

            2.   Is he in positive nitrogen balance? *No***
                  Base your answer by using this chart data: **<u>Nitrogen Intake</u>** *= 21 g/24 hours*
                  Initially, it appears that Bobby is in nitrogen balance. However, actually, due to very high loss of protein from his burn injury and his hypermetabolic state, he is in severe negative nitrogen balance. The UUN only measures what is lost through the urine. Normally, an additional 4g of protein loss is added to the UUN loss based on normal nonurine loss of proteins. Bobby's additional loss would be significantly higher.

      C.   **Weight Status**
            Bobby weighed <u>*155*</u> pounds prior to admission. Currently he weighs <u>*138*</u> pounds. This represents an <u>*11*</u> percent weight loss.

            Is this percent of weight loss significant? If yes, in what way? *Yes. More than a 10% weight loss is considered significant for malnutrition.*

D. **Protein Measurement**
  1. **Visceral Protein**
     a. Bobby's serum albumin is *1.9* g/dL. What is the significance of this value to Bobby's nutritional status? *His intravascular oncotic pressure will be low due to lack of protein. This will allow fluids to leave his intravascular space and move into the extravascular spaces. It also represents a severe level of malnutrition.*

E. **Physical Assessment for Protein and Protein-Calorie Malnutrition:**
  The following are typical clinical findings consistent with protein-calorie malnutrition. Which could be assess in Bobby's situation? Does he have any of these present?

System	Able to Assess	Present (Yes/No)
Integumentary:		
-Decreased subcu fat	No	
-Flaky, dry skin	No	
-Shedding of hair No		
Musculoskeletal:		
-Muscle wasting	Yes	Yes
-Edema present	Yes	Yes
Cardiovascular:		
-Evidence of dec. Yes C.O.	Insuff. evidence via available data	
Evidence of lack of healing:	Yes	Yes

F. **What conclusions can you draw from the nutritional data you have gathered here?**
  Bobby cannot be assessed based on his integumentary data. He is in a hypermetabolic state. His weight loss is most significant sign available.

G. **Examine Bobby's Serum Electrolytes:**

Electrolyte	Normal Range	Bobby's Value
Sodium	135 - 145 mEq/L *128*	
Chloride	96 - 106 mEq/L	*94*
Potassium	3.5 - 5.5 mEq/L	*2.9*
Total Calcium	4.3 - 5.5 mEq/L	*4.1*
Phosphorus	3.0 - 4.5 mg/dL	*1.8*
Magnesium	1.5 - 2.2 mEq/L	*1.2*

  1. **Why are they abnormal?** *Significant fluid shifts occur, altering circulating blood volume. Fluid as well as electrolytes move into the interstitial spaces due to damaged capillaries and fluid and electrolytes are also lost at the sites of the burn.*
  2. **Which one(s) should be addressed FIRST? Why?** *Priority should be placed on those electrolyte deficiencies that are the most dangerous to Bobby -- His potassium and his calcium.*
  3. **Does Bobby currently exhibit any clinical manifestations that are consistent with any of these electrolyte deficits?** *Confusion is the most overt. He is not showing cardiac problems at this time and other manifestations are masked by his critical state.*

H.   Is Bobby in a hypermetabolic state?   If he is, when will it cease to exist?
       Yes. It will exist until his burn wounds have all been resolved either through healing (partial thickness burns) or skin grafting (full thickness burns).

I.   **Immunocompetence Assessment**
       A.   **Which of the following critical cues suggesting immunocompetence problems does Bobby exhibit, it any?**

Critical Cue	Present (Y/N)
Fever	*Yes*
Poor wound healing	*Yes*
Abnormal CBC with Diff.	*Yes*
Abnormal coagulation studies	*No data*
Recurrent, prolonged, or severe infections	*Yes*
Secondary infections	*Yes*
Immunosuppressive drug therapy	*No*
Other at-risk factors	*Yes*

       B.   **Total Lymphocyte Count (TLC)**
              1.   Examine the most recent CBC with diff. Using the given formula, determine the TLC.

$$TLC = \frac{\% \text{ Lymphocytes} \times WBC}{100}$$

[Bobby's % lymphs = 9%, WBC =12,000:]
$$TLC = \frac{9.0 \times 12,000}{100} = 1,080$$

              2.   Bobby's TLC is currently *1,080.*

       C.   **What do the available data tell you about Bobby's immunocomptence status?**
              His TLC indicates a moderate immunodeficiency at this time. However it will, most likely, continue to deteriorate to the severe range due to his hypermetabolic state and high loss of protein.
       D.   **What is the relationship between Bobby's malnutrition status and his immuno-competence status?**
              As his malnutrition becomes more severe, so will his immunodeficient state. This is due to the composition of the immune system which is primarily protein.

3.   **Nursing Implications**
       A.   **List 5 nursing diagnoses that would be appropriate based on this data base:**
              1.   *High risk for injury r/t electrolyte imbalances*
              2.   *Alt. in nutrition: less than body requirements r/t hypermetabolic state*
              3.   *Infection r/t extensive loss of skin integrity*
              4.   *High risk for decreased cardiac output r/t significant loss of intravascular fluids secondary to low oncotic pressure (low serum albumin levels)*
              5.   *High risk for fluid volume deficit*
       B.   **What would be the major expected patient outcomes for Bobby based on the nursing diagnoses you have developed?** *[WNL = within normal limits]*
              1.   *Electrolytes WNL*
              2.   *Weight WNL for age, height & weight*
              3.   *CBC WNL*
              4.   *Serum albumin, BUN, Creatinine WNL*
              5.   *Absence of signs of decreased cardiac output (specify)*

C.   **List 5 collaborative interventions that you would anticipate based on your nursing diagnoses:**
1. *Serial laboratory data (Electrolytes, Osmolality, CBC, BUN, Creatinine, UUN)*
2. *Electrolyte and fluid replacement*
3. *Tube feeding orders*
4. *Antibiotic therapy*
5. *Hemodynamic lines and monitoring*
6. *Cardiac monitoring*

D.   **List 5 independent nursing interventions that your would anticipate, based on your nursing diagnoses:**
1. *Monitor for clinical manifestations of electrolyte imbalances (specify)*
2. *Monitor for clinical manifestations of decreased cardiac output (specify)*
3. *Monitor for clinical manifestations of infection (specify)*
4. *Daily weights during fluid shifts. Weekly weights following fluid shifts.*
5. *Vital signs (frequency based on stability of Bobby)*
6. *Monitor for therapeutic and nontherapeutic effects of tube feedings*

Problem Solving Exercise
The Case of Mike Brady

Directions: Appoint a scribe to be in charge of writing necessary information on index cards in Tasks #1, #3, #5, #7, and #8 for each group. Appoint a speaker to represent each group during the interactions.

INITIAL FRAME

Mike Brady, 15 years old, was brought to the hospital by friends after a dirt bike crash. He was alert and oriented in the Emergency Department but complained of severe left thigh pain. His admitting vital signs were: B/P = 90/60, HR = 122, R =28. His skin was warm, pale, and dry. He had abrasions to both knees and a deformed left thigh with bone ends protruding.

****

Task #1: [The scribe should have one index card]
> Using the index card provided, develop a list of at least four additional pieces of data relating to Mike's mechanism of injury that would be helpful in anticipating the severity of his injuries.

Task #2:
> Should Mike's deformed thigh be splinted during the primary or secondary trauma assessment? Justify your response.

****

Mike is taken to the operating suite where his fracture site was irrigated and debrided. The left femur fracture was stabilized internally with an intermedullary nail. He is transferred to you from the post-anesthesia recovery unit.
****

Task #3: [Scribe should have an index card]
> List three factors that influences Mike's wound healing abilities based on his injury event.

Task #4:
> What two medical problems is Mike at risk for during the third trauma mortality peak?

****

It is now day 15 post admission for Mike. During your morning assessment, you position Mike on his side and note that he has developed an area of breakdown on his coccyx. His vital signs are B/P 120/82, HR 88, R 16, T 100.8 oral. He has lost 20 pounds since admission. Mike has been nauseated and he has not been taking fluids well for the past several days. His thigh incision is red, with light yellow, thick drainage. He has gone to Physical Therapy twice but complains of fatigue and pain. He refused to go today. He has a productive cough with white sputum.
****

Task #5:

Develop a problem list and cluster these problems into appropriate nursing diagnoses.

PROBLEM LIST:

NURSING DIAGNOSES

Task #6:

Since Mike has developed skin breakdown plus he has a surgical incision, we know that impaired skin integrity is an appropriate diagnosis. Complete the nursing diagnosis statement and list EPOs in the space provided.

Impaired skin integrity r/t:

EPO: Mike will have no evidence of further breakdown AEB:

Task #7:

What type of collaborative and independent nursing interventions will you include in your plan to successfully maintain or attain your EPOs? Keep in mind that your interventions will need to include how you will measure each of the EPOs.

COLLABORATIVE INTERVENTIONS:

INDEPENDENT NURSING INTERVENTIONS:

Task #8:
    List 5 additional complications Mike is at risk of experiencing because of his decreased mobility.

[This completes the case of Mike Brady]

The Case of Mike Brady:
A Problem Solving Exercise
Instructor Guide

Directions: Appoint a scribe to be in charge of writing necessary information on index cards in Tasks #1, #3, #5, #7, and #8 for each group. Appoint a speaker to represent each group during the interactions.

INITIAL FRAME

Mike Brady, 15 years old, was brought to the hospital by friends after a dirt bike crash. He was alert and oriented in the Emergency Department but complained of severe left thigh pain. His admitting vital signs were: B/P = 90/60, HR = 122, R =28. His skin was warm, pale, and dry. He had abrasions to both knees and a deformed left thigh with bone ends protruding.

****

Task #1: [The scribe should have one index card]
Using the index card provided, develop a list of at least four additional pieces of data relating to Mike's mechanism of injury that would be helpful in anticipating the severity of his injuries.

1. Was he wearing a helmet?
2. What speed was he traveling?
3. What surface did he hit/land upon?
4. Did he lose consciousness at the scene?
5. Has he been using drugs or alcohol?

****

Task #2: Should Mike's deformed thigh be splinted during the primary or secondary trauma assessment ? Justify your response.

1. *Primary survey: Only if his thigh is actively bleeding and the degree of blood loss could compromise his circulation.*

2. *Secondary survey: Since it is potentially (versus actual) life threatening at this point, his thigh should be splinted during the secondary survey. Supporting data: B/P 90/60, HR = 122 could be related to sympathetic nervous system response related to pain, anxiety, or blood loss.*

****

Mike is taken to the operating suite where his fracture site was irrigated and debrided. The left femur fracture was stabilized internally with an intermedullary nail. He is transferred to you from the post-anesthesia recovery unit.
****

Task #3: [Scribe should have an index card]
List three factors that influences Mike's wound healing abilities based on his injury event.
1.hypoperfusion r/t blood loss during surgery and at time of injury
2.hypermetabolism r/t injury response (requires greater protein)
3.high infection potential r/t dirty wound
4.decreased peripheral perfusion r/t decreased mobility/bedrest

Task #4: What two medical problems is Mike at risk for during the third trauma mortality peak?
1 . MODS or sepsis r/t bacterial contamination of wound, decreased perfusion
2. renal failure r/t myoglobin release due to long bone fracture

****

It is now day 15 post admission for Mike. During your morning assessment, you position Mike on his side and note that he has developed an area of breakdown on his coccyx. His vital signs are B/P 120/82, HR 88, R 16, T 100.8 oral. He has lost 20 pounds since admission. Mike has been nauseated and he has not been taking fluids well for the past several days. His thigh incision is red, with light yellow, thick drainage. He has gone to Physical Therapy twice but complains of fatigue and pain. He refused to go today. He has a productive cough with white sputum.

****

Task #5: Develop a problem list and cluster these problems into appropriate nursing diagnoses.

PROBLEM LIST:

1. Fever
2. Yellow drainage from incision
3. Productive cough
4. Weight loss of 20 pounds since admission
5. Pain
6. Decreased mobility
7. Skin breakdown

NURSING DIAGNOSES

1. Infection
2. Alteration in Nutrition: Less than body requirements
3. Impaired Skin Integrity
4. Impaired Physical Mobility
5. Pain

Task #6: Since Mike has developed skin breakdown plus he has a surgical incision, we know that impaired skin integrity is an appropriate diagnosis. Complete the nursing diagnosis statement and list EPOs in the space provided.

Impaired Skin Integrity r/t: _increased pressure on bony prominences, weight loss, and surgical procedure as evidenced by yellow thick, incision drainage, sacral abrasion ._

EPO: Mike will have:
a) no further skin breakdown
b) gradual reduction in redness and swelling at incision site
c) serosanguinous drainage
d) presence of granulation tissue

Task #7: What type of collaborative and independent nursing interventions will you include in your plan to successfully maintain or attain your EPOs? Keep in mind that your interventions will need to include how you will measure each of the EPOs.

COLLABORATIVE INTERVENTIONS: *(partial list of possible orders)*
1. Dressing change per physician order
2. Wound culture prior to antibiotic administration
3. Antibiotic Administration

INDEPENDENT NURSING INTERVENTIONS: (*partial list of possible interventions*)

1. *Decrease stress to incision line and coccyx area*
    a) *turn patient q hour*
    b) *make sure incision dressing is secured to prevent rubbing q dressing change*
    c) *have patient shift weight q 30 minutes*
    d) *apply eggcrate mattress*
    e) *elevate coccyx off the bed (may require an order for a specialized support surface)*

2. *Increase perfusion to wounds*
    a) *heat lamp to coccyx 15 minutes q 4 hours*
    b) *encourage ambulation/weight bearing per physician and PT protocol*

3. *Promote nutrition*
    a) *daily weight*
    b) *avoid ambulating patient prior to meals*
    c) *offer high protein snacks*

Task #8: List 5 additional complications Mike is at risk of experiencing because of his decreased mobility.

1. *Pneumonia r/t stasis of pulmonary secretions*
2. *Deep vein thrombosis r/t local irritation of vessels secondary to injury and venous stasis*
3. *Constipation r/t decreased fluid intake, decreased peristalsis, supine position*
4. *Renal calculi/UTI r/t decreased fluid intake, hypercalcemia secondary to decreased bone stress*
5. *Stress ulcers r/t decreased nutritional intake and increased gastric acid secretion*

[This completes the case of Mike Brady]

Clinical Focus: Injury

Student name: _____ Date: _____

Patient initials: _____. Age:_____ Gender:_____ Admission date:_____

Admission diagnosis: _____

Surgeries/Procedures: _____

****

[Note: The patient assigned should have experienced an injury event.]

Assessment

1. Document any demographic information potentially related to injury outcomes (eg. age, education, gender, etc).

2. What factors are present that mediate the injury response?

   Address drugs/medications, past medical conditions, and anatomic and physiologic factors.

3. What signs were discovered in the emergency care setting that indicated injuries were present?

Analysis

4. What forces were involved in producing the injury? (e.g., acceleration, deceleration, shearing, yawing, tumbling, etc.).

5. What injuries are present due to these forces?

6. What are your priority nursing diagnoses?

7. For which type of trauma sequelae is your patient most at risk? Why?

Physical Examination

8. What signs are present that suggest complications may be present?

Interventions

9. What nursing interventions are you performing to prevent complications?

10. What nursing interventions are you performing to help the patient compensate for the complications?

PART VIII

LIFE SPAN: SPECIAL NEEDS

Part VIII. Table of Contents

PART VIII. LIFE SPAN: SPECIAL NEEDS

Take Home Cases (THC)

The Acutely Ill Pediatric Patient (Module 32)   303
The Acutely Ill Obstetric Patient (Module 33)   306
The Acutely Ill Elderly Patient (Module 34)   309

Case Studies

The Case of Mary Case   311
The Case of Baby TJ   318
The Case of Amanda   325

Take Home Case
Module 32: Acutely Ill Pediatric Patient

Student name:_____   Date:_____

DIRECTIONS:
        Using the appropriate reading assignment, complete the following questions or statements using complete sentences.
****

Section: Ventilation

1.   What are the three functional types of ventilation problems in childhood?

2.   What signs indicate acute respiratory failure in children?

Section: Perfusion

3.   How does a child increase cardiac output?

4.   What causes life threatening dysrhythmias in children?

5.   What rate of infusion is used for rapid fluid resuscitation in children?

Section: Cognition/Perception

6.   What signs indicate meningeal irritation?

7.   What metabolic abnormality precipitates seizures in children?

Section: Metabolism/Thermoregulation

8.   Bobby Jo weighs 10 Kg. Calculate his daily maintenance fluids.

9.   Bobby Jo weighed 12 Kg. prior to becoming ill. Calculate fluid replacement needs.

Section: Immunocompetence

10. List five assessment cues that indicate possible immunosuppression.

Section: Psychosocial Factors

11. How do toddlers behave when separated from their parents?

12. Which developmental age would react favorably to using band aids over puncture wounds?

> infant
> toddler
> preschool
> school age
> adolescent

Take Home Case
Module 32: Acutely Ill Pediatric Patient
Instructor Guide

1. obstructive lung disease
   restrictive lung disease
   primary ineffective gas transfer

2. tachypnea initially followed by bradypnea
   strider
   wheezing, grunting
   retractions
   nasal flaring
   use of accessory muscle
   tachycardia leading to bradycardia
   pale, dusky, cyanotic
   $SpO_2 < 95\%$

3. increases the heart rate

4. hypoxemia and acidosis

5. 20cc/Kg

6. Kernig's and Brudzinski's signs
   irritability

7. hypoglycemia

8. 10 x 100 = 1000cc/24 hours

9. 12Kg - 10Kg = 2Kg
   2Kg/12Kg =.16
   % weight loss = 16%
   10ml/Kg x 16 = 160cc fluid loss
   160cc fluid loss x 12Kg = 1920 total fluid deficit
   1920 = 1000 = 2920cc replacement

10. refer to Table 32-32 (Module 32)

11. temper tantrums
    uncooperative behavior

12. preschool

Take Home Case
Module 33: Acutely Ill Obstetric Patient

Student name: _____   Date:_____

DIRECTIONS:
        Using the appropriate reading assignment complete the following questions or statements using complete sentences.
****

Section one:
1. What effect does pregnancy have on the cardiovascular septum?

Section two:
2. What is the 3rd stage of labor?

3. List factors that interfere with a nonstress test:

4. Which of the following are /is an omnious sign?

        ()   accelerations
        ()   early decelerations
        ()   variable decelerations
        ()   late decelerations

Section three:
5. What are the signs of an amniotic fluid embolus?

Section four:
6. A patient who has had a history of hypertension and exhibits hypertension during pregnancy is classified as

      _____.

7. What criteria are needed for a diagnosis of pre-eclampsia?

Section Five:
8. In patients with HELLP syndrome, delivery is postponed if possible until fetal maturity is achieved.
        <u>True or False</u> (circle one)

Section six:
9. A patient with sudden onset of painless bleeding in the second or third trimester is probably experiencing

      _____.

10. When does post partum hemorrhage most frequently occur?

Section seven:

11. In pregnancy, greater blood loss must occur for clinical signs of shock to be present.

   True or False (circle one)

Section eight:

12. Which organs are most frequently affected by blunt trauma during pregnancy?

Section nine:

13. The best test to get an average of circulating blood sugar for 4 to 6 weeks prior is _____.

14. If a diabetic mother experiences pre-term labor, what problem may occur from use of beta-agonist drugs and steroids?

Section ten:

15. List five symptoms of pre-term labor:

Section eleven:

16. What are fetal effects from cocaine abuse?

Section twelve:

17. What position should the mother be placed in emergency delivery with a prolapsed cord?

Section thirteen:

18. An infant with acrocyanosis should receive high levels of oxygen.

   True or False (circle one)

Take Home Case
Module 33: Acutely Ill Obstetric Patient
Instructor Guide

1. increased stroke volume and cardiac output
   B/P decreases initially then returns to normal
   reduced SVR
   increased renal blood flow

2. delivery of the infant to delivery of the placenta
3. cigarette smoking, fetal sleep patterns
4. late decelerations
5. acute respiratory distress
   chills
   shivering
   sweating
   pink, frothy sputum

6. chronic hypertension
7. increase in B/P by at least 30mm systolic or 15mm diastolic
   edema
   proteinuria

8. False
9. placenta previa
10. one hour after delivery
11. True
12. genitourinary tract, abdomen (liver, spleen, uterus)
13. hemoglobin A/C test
14. hyperglycemia
15. uterine contractions
    cramps
    backache
    pelvic pressure
    increased vaginal D/C
    bloody vaginal D/C

16. abruptio placenta
    pre-term
    decreased fetal weight
    abnormalities of the GU, cardiovascular and CNS systems

17. knee-chest, bed in Trendelenburg position

18. False

Take Home Case
Module 34: Acutely Ill Elderly Patients

Student name: _____ Date:_____

DIRECTIONS:
        Using the appropriate reading assignment, complete the following questions or statements using complete sentences.
****

Section one:
1.   List five age related physiologic changes.

Section two:
2.   Define "functional decline":

Section three:
3.   Cognitive impairment may first present in changes in _____.

Section four:
5.   What complications may occur in the mechanical ventilated elderly patient?

Section five:
6.   Changes in ST-T waves indicate ischemia in the elderly patient.
        <u>True or False</u>

Section six:
7.   What differentiates dementia from depression and delirium?

Section seven:
8.   List signs of infection in the elderly patient.

Section eight:
9.   Why are headache and vomiting not signs of increased ICP in the elderly?

Section nine:
10. Why is the half life of anesthetic agents prolonged in the elderly?

Take Home Case
Module 34: Acutely Ill Elderly Patients
Instructor Guide

1. See Table 34-1

2. Recent difficulty or the inability to perform tasks that are necessary or desirable for independent living.

3. Instrumental activities of daily living

4. acute renal failure
   dependent or increased renin levels to keep renal perfuse adequate

5. Nosocomial pneumonia
   CHF

6. False

7. Dementia is insidious, progressive, and irreversible

8. change in mental status

   functional decline

   history of a fall

   hypothermia

   altered blood glucose

   acidosis

   tachycardia

9. Because age related cerebral atrophy allows for great increases in ICP before signs occur. When the occur, cranial nerve deficits and change in LOC are common.

10. decreased total body water
    decreased vascular tone
    sluggish circulation

Case Study
The Case of Mary Case: An Acutely Ill Obstetric Patient

Mrs. Case is 30 years old, 7 months pregnant, and was involved in a motor vehicle crash. She was the restrained driver. She was transported by ambulance to the Emergency Department (ED) of the hospital where you work in the ICU. You have been pulled to work in the ED because they are short staffed. You are assigned to care for Mrs. Case. Mrs. Case has just arrived and the paramedics give you the following report.

Recent History

Mrs. Case had no loss of consciousness at the crash scene. Her lap belt was on. Her blood pressure in the field was 80/60. The paramedics started 2 large bore IVs with Lactated Ringers. Her blood pressure on arrival is 110/70.

Past History

Mrs. Case is Gravida II, Para I. She has a 3 year old child at home. Normal pregnancy with first child. No problems thus far in present pregnancy. She wants a tubal ligation after this child. Past medical history is non-significant.

The Initial Appraisal

You quickly note the following upon entering her patient care area and seeing her on the stretcher:

General appearance: Mrs. Case is pale. Her respirations are labored. She is receiving 40% oxygen per face mask. She keeps asking about her baby. C-collar is in place and the patient is laying supine on a backboard. Her abdomen is gravid.

Signs of distress: You note that her respirations are rapid. She tries to move on the backboard and is moaning.

Other: She is in sinus tachycardia without ectopy on the cardiac monitor. IVs are infusing in both antecubital veins. IV sites are without signs of irritation and infiltration.

Systemic Bedside Assessment

Head and Neck

Mrs. Case is oriented to person, place and year. Her Glasgow Coma Scale is 15. Her neck veins are flat in the supine position. There are multiple minor lacerations on her face with glass present. No active bleeding is noted.

Chest

Pulmonary status: Vesicular breaths sounds auscultated on the right. Breath sounds absent on the left. Her respiratory rate is currently 36/minute. Her breathing is moderately labored and shallow. No sub-cutaneous air noted.

Cardiac status: S_1 and S_2 are auscultated. No murmur is noted. Her apical rate is regular at 118/minute.

Abdomen

Bowel sounds are absent. Abdomen has multiple abrasions and contusions. A 4 cm ecchymotic area is noted in the RLQ. Abdomen is rigid and tender on palpation. Fetal heart sounds 110 by doppler.

Pelvis/Genitalia

A contusion is noted over the right ramus, approximately 10 mm in diameter. Swollen labia with bright red bloody drainage is present.

Extremities:

+2 peripheral pulses are assessed. Her capillary refill is greater than three seconds. Nail beds are pale-pink. Skin is cool and dry.

Vital Signs:

Currently: BP = 100/70; P = 120, regular; R = 36/minute, somewhat labored; T = 98.8 (o).

Her ranges over the hour:

BP = $\frac{80 - 110}{60 - 70}$, P = 90 - 120/minute, R = 20 - 36/minute

Psychosocial Assessment:

Husband drove himself to the hospital and is waiting in the ED lobby. Very concerned about his wife's and child's status. Mrs. Case does not work outside the home. She is very active in church. Rarely drinks alcohol. Does not smoke.

Significant Labs and other tests:

SERUM:

WBC: 31.14

Hemoglobin: 9

Hematocrit: 24.8

Glucose: 236

BUN: 9

Creatinine : 0.8

Electrolytes: Within normal ranges

URINE:

1 to 5 RBCs, Negative protein and glucose

Portable Chest X-ray:

Left pneumothorax with left hemidiaphragm. Left rib fractures 9-10.

Intake and Output :

Intake = 5000 cc LR

Output = 100 cc

Weight:

Admission = 165 pounds (per husband report)

Arterial Blood Gases:

On 40% face mask: pH = 7.32, PCO_2 = 49, PO_2 = 76, HCO_3 = 28, SaO_2 = 88%.

Physician Orders:

Oxygen @ 100% per face mask.

NPO. N/G to LWS.

Urinary catheter to BSD.

Type and Cross for 8 units of packed RBCs, give 2 units ASAP.

IVF LR wide open to keep systolic B/P > 100.

Continuous monitoring of fetal heart tones.

Chest tube to 20 cm suction

Medications:

Keflin 1 gm IV now

Metronidazole 500 mg IV now

Anesthesia pre op for OR

The Case of Mary Case: Study Guide

Admitting Diagnosis:_____

Age:_____

Note: The Case of Mary Case is a reality based case presentation. The data available may show evidence of multiple problem areas. The focus of today's case study, however, is on trauma in pregnancy. Thus, most of the questions in this exercise will center around consideration of her pregnant state.

1.   **Past Medical and Social History:**

2.   **Events leading to admission:**

3.   **Initial Appraisal**
      What abnormal data did you collect from your initial appraisal of Mary

4.   **Based on your initial appraisal, what priority assessment clusters will you immediately focus in on?**

5.   **In what sequence would you implement the physician orders based on your assessment clusters?**

6.   **Based on your data clusters/problems, what do you now believe is/are Mrs. Case's acute medical problem(s)?**

7. **Based on your data clusters/problems, what do you see as your priority nursing diagnoses?** Place a check mark in the provided space for those diagnoses that appropriate. Complete the nursing diagnosis statement and list the outcome criteria in the space provided.

    1. _____**Impaired Gas Exchange R/T**_____.

        The patient will maintain effective gas exchange clearance, as evidenced by:
        a)

        b)

        c)

        d)

    2. _____**Ineffective Breathing Patterns R/T**_____.

        The patient will maintain an effective breathing pattern, evidenced by:
        a)

        b)

        c)

        d)

    3._____**Fluid Volume Deficit R/T**_____.

        The patient will maintain adequate fluid volume, as evidenced by:
        a)

        b)

        c)

        d)

    4. Is there an actual or potential nursing diagnosis that might apply to Mrs. Case's fetus's condition? If so, state the nursing diagnosis.

8. **List appropriate _independent_ nursing interventions that address the nursing diagnoses you have chosen.**

The Case of Mary Case Study Guide
Instructor Guide

Admitting
Diagnosis:_____

Age:_____

Note: The Case of Mary Case is a reality based case presentation. The data available may show evidence of multiple problem areas. The focus of today's case study, however, is on trauma in pregnancy. Thus, most of the questions in this exercise will center around consideration of her pregnant state.

1.   **Past Medical and Social History:**
        gravida II, para I
        no problems in this pregnancy
        well child at home
        wants tubal ligation post delivery
        husband supportive
        church is potential support system

2.   **Events leading to admission:**
        MVC
        restrained driver
        prehospital hypotension supported by IV Lactated Ringers

3.   **Initial Appraisal**
        What abnormal data did you collect from your initial appraisal of Mary
        Respirations labored and rapid even with oxygen administration, absent breath sounds on left
        is in sinus tachycardia, she is pale, lying supine

4.   **Based on your initial appraisal, what priority assessment clusters will you immediately focus in on?**

        Ventilation cluster:
                -absent breath sounds on the left
                -labored, shallow, rapid respirations
                -respiratory acidosis
                -ruptured diaphragm, left pneumothorax, on chest film
                -supine, high risk for aspiration

        Perfusion cluster:
                -hypotension especially for pregnant state
                -rigid, tender abdomen
                -bright red vaginal bleeding
                -absent fetal heart tones
                -ecchymotic area RLQ
                -supine, high risk for decreased venous return

        Note: This is a good time to discuss hemodilution in pregnancy. Compare Ms. Case's hempglobin and hematocrit values with normal values for pregnancy (For example, her hemoglobin is 9 compared to 10-13 for pregnancy: therefore, she may have blood loss. Her hematocrit is 24.8 compared to 32-42, indicating hemoconcentration.).

5.   **In what sequence would you implement the physician orders based on your assessment clusters?**
  1)   -change oxygen rate 40% to 100%
  2)   -prepare for chest tube insertion
  3)   -insert NG tube (maintain airway patency)
  4)   -confirm type and crossmatch has been drawn with earlier labs or obtain sample
  5)   -insert urinary catheter
  6)   -administer medications

6.   **Based on your data clusters/problems, what do you now believe is/are Mrs. Case's acute medical problem(s)?**
  -pneumothorax
  -ruptured diaphragm
  -abruptio placenta vs. ruptured uterus
  -possible fetal death
  -potential other abdominal organ laceration due to blunt trauma

7.   **Based on your data clusters/problems, what do you see as your priority nursing diagnoses?** Place a check mark in the provided space for those diagnoses that appropriate. Complete the nursing diagnosis statement and list the outcome criteria in the space provided.

  1. _____**Impaired Gas Exchange R/T**_____.

      The patient will maintain effective gas exchange clearance, as evidenced by:
      a) *no respiratory acidosis*
      b) *no change in level of responsiveness*
      c) *no cyanosis*
      d) *oxygen saturation WNL*

  2. _____**Ineffective Breathing Patterns R/T**_____.

      The patient will maintain an effective breathing pattern, evidenced by:
      a) *no accessory muscle use*
      b) *no fatigue from ventilation*
      c) *vesicular breath sounds auscultated in right lung fields*

  3._____**Fluid Volume Deficit R/T**_____.

      The patient will maintain adequate fluid volume, as evidenced by:
      a) *urine output of 1ml/kg/hr*
      b) *jugular veins filled*
      c) *CVP within normal limits (if measured)*
      d) *no further decrease in blood pressure*

  4.   Is there an actual or potential nursing diagnosis that might apply to Mrs. Case's fetus's condition? If so, state the nursing diagnosis.
      High risk for injury R/T hypoxia AEB bradycardia
      Anticipatory Grieving R/Potential fetal intrauterine damage or death

8.   **List appropriate __independent__ nursing interventions that address the nursing diagnoses you have chosen.**

  1. place wedge under right side of backboard
  2. prime blood tubing and have blood warmer available
  3. monitor for uterine contractions, fetal movement, FHT
  4. suction PRN

5. *measure fundal height*
6. *measure vaginal bleeding*

Case Study
The Case of Baby TJ
A Patient with a Pulmonary Problem

Baby TJ is a 10 weeks old male. His admission diagnosis is prematurity, and Infant Respiratory Distress Syndrome. TJ has been in the neonatal ICU since birth. He was born at 30 weeks gestation, weighing 1450 grams. His mother is 28 years old, G_3 P_2 A_1. At birth, TJ's APGARS were 5, 6. He was intubated at birth, initially requiring high ventilator settings (100% oxygenated at times). His patent ductus arteriosus opened on day three and was treated with indomethacin. His weight gain has been sporadic with occasional periods of feeding intolerance and frequent emesis. He is slowly being weaned from a mechanical ventilator. He continues to have mild to moderate respiratory distress with CO_2 retention and variable oxygenation.

TJ's family is very supportive. His father works days at a local pharmacy. His mother is not currently working and stays at the hospital almost continuously. The nurse notices that she appears fatigued. They also have a 5 year old son who is currently staying with relatives in a nearby town. They are actively involved in a local church which has been very supportive. While eager to take TJ home, they are very concerned about his daily care needs and the possibility of his dying at home. They have satisfactory health insurance.

Initial Nursing Assessment

VS: BP = 82/58, P = 168, R = 64/min., T = 98.8 (A). Weight = 1970 g, head circumference 32.5 cm

Neurological: TJ is alert and responsive. His fontanels are flat. He calms when his mother rocks or pats him on his back. He is calmest when tightly bundled. He sucks on a pacifier. He is irritable but in no obvious distress.

Pulmonary: TJ is very pale. His skin is warm and slightly diaphoretic. He becomes cyanotic with agitation. Breath sounds are equal bilaterally with coarse crackles (rales) auscultated bilaterally. An occasional expiratory wheeze is also noted. He has moderate substernal and intercostal retractions. His secretions are small to moderate in quantity and white during suctioning (every 4 hours).

Cardiovascular: No audible murmur is noted.

Gastrointestinal: TJ has been having difficulty tolerating his oral feedings. He has a poor suck reflex and uncoordinated swallowing. He also tires quickly from feeding activities. Currently, he is receiving nutrition via PO and NG feedings, taking 5 - 15 mL per feeding. Unless he receives his feedings very slowly, he vomits. During feedings, he requires increased oxygen concentrations. His abdomen is soft and flat with a stable abdominal circumference. Mild to moderate edema is noted and his neck veins are distended. Bowel sounds are present. No visible loops are noted. He has 4 - 6 bowel movements daily which are yellow. He has bilateral inguinal hernias which are reducible.

Genitourinary: TJ is Lasix dependent. His urinary output is 3-4 cc/kg/hr with a specific gravity of 1.012. His Dextrostix = 90. His genitalia are normal for his age.

Musculoskeletal: TJ moves all extremities. He develops increase respiratory distress with activity. Muscle tone is normal.

Medical Team Findings and Progress Notes

1. Premature infant with Respiratory distress
2. Ventilator dependent; difficult to wean; attempting course of steroids.

3.   Bilateral hernias continue to be reducible; postpone surgery until condition stabilizes.

4.   Lasix dependent. Requiring potassium replacements. Fluid restricted.

5.   Poor weight gain. Polycose added to feedings.

CURRENT STATUS REPORT

Intake: 260 mL or Similac 24 with Iron and 15 mL of polycose.

Output: 210 mL with specific gravity of 1.014. Feeding tube residual of 28 mL -- returned. Four bowel movements, yellow and seedy in small to moderate amounts.

Breath sounds: Equal, with crackles. Moderate retractions. Small amount of white secretions.

Neurologic: Irritable, awake and alert with care.

Vital Signs: P = 172, R = 58

Chest X-ray: cardiomegaly, hyperexpanded lungs, and diffuse infiltrates.

Current abnormal labs:

    ABG: $pH = 7.31$, $PCO_2 = 54$, $SaO_2 = > 90\%$ at rest but $<90\%$ with activity and deep sleep

    K+:   3.2

    Cl: 96

    Theophylline level = 7.2

CURRENT MEDICAL ORDERS

1.   NICU protocol

2.   Ventilator settings:

                Rate: 8 breaths per minute

                PAP/PEEP = 20/3

                $FiO_2 = 42\%$ (keep saturations > 90)

3.   Labs: CBC, Hct, Na, and K every day

                  Theophylline level every Monday

4.   Feeding: Similac 24 with Iron at 24 cc every 2 hours. 2.5 mL polycose every other feeding

5.   Medications:

    Theophylline

    Aldactone

    Decadron

    KCl

    MVI

    Feosol

    PRN Medications: Lasix, additional KCl, and Terbutaline

The Case of Baby TJ Study Guide

I. **VENTILATION**

    A.   Examine TJ's respiratory status. Does he have a restrictive, obstructive or combination of both airway problem? Defend your choice.

    B.   The scenario describes a pattern of increasing hypoxemia with agitation. What type of nursing measures can be taken to minimize this oxygenation problem?

    C.   As a newborn, you would be most concerned if TJ developed a respiratory rate of
        >_____.

    D.   Why is tachypnea a priority assessment in the very young? In addition to rate, what other nursing assessments are important in this age group?

    E.   The module lists criteria used in children to discriminate between two types of respiratory failure: Type I and Type II. Which does TJ have? Is it consistent with the probable diagnosis? [refer to page 748]

II. **PERFUSION**

TJ's blood pressure is 82/58, his pulse is 168 and respirations are 64/minute. At 3 days post birth, his ductus arteriosus opened.

A.   A.   What is the clinical significance of his patent ductus arteriosus?

            B.   Examine TJ's blood pressure and pulse and respirations. Interpret these values based on his age.

C.   Is there evidence of decreased peripheral tissue perfusion?

III.   FLUIDS

    A.   The nurse is assessing for the signs of dehydration in TJ. What would be assessed in a neonate?

    B.   What kind of intravenous solution support would you anticipate to help maintain TJ's perfusion?

    C.   If TJ weighs approximately 2 Kg, his daily maintenance fluid needs would be _____ mL.

    D.   What interventions can the nurse take to reduce TJ's risk of infection?

[If there is sufficient time, the teacher might want to explore the psychosocial aspects of this problem (i.e. the parent's fears, financial implications, etc.]

The Case of Baby TJ Study Guide
Instructor Guide

I.   VENTILATION

A.   **Examine TJ's respiratory status. Does he have a restrictive, obstructive or combination of both airway problem? Defend your choice.**

One would argue that he has a primary restrictive disorder with some obstructive involvement.

TJ has strong evidence to support a restrictive problem. Critical cues available based on the scenario include: Immaturity by history, hypoxemia, the presence of crackles (rales) on auscultation, cyanosis with agitation, probable decreased lung compliance as evidenced by requiring high ventilator settings, and his chest x-ray showed diffuse bilateral infiltrates. These are also consistent with the existing medical diagnosis of Infant Respiratory Distress Syndrome (Hyaline Membrane Disease) which is associated with massive atelectasis, another restrictive pulmonary problem.

He also has evidence to support some degree of obstructive disease, as evidenced by respiratory acidosis (per ABG) which indicates alveolar hypoventilation. His chest x-ray showed hyperexpanded lungs. Finally, his occasional expiratory wheeze reflects airway constriction and/or bronchospasm, both obstructive airway problems.

B.   **The scenario describes a pattern of increasing hypoxemia with agitation. What type of nursing measures can be taken to minimize this oxygenation problem?**

Take measures to increase oxygen supply and reduce oxygen demand. Increasing TJ's oxygen concentration during periods of stimulation and maintaining airway clearance through close monitoring and PRN suctioning are the two most important actions to increase supply. Increasing the head of the bed may enhance breathing by keeping the abdominal organs from pushing on the diaphragm.

Decreasing oxygen can be accomplished by minimizing activities that cause a state of agitation such as painful procedures. Balance his need to suck with his need to rest by continuing a combination of short sucking periods on bottle and primary nutrition via tube feedings. Since his carbon dioxide levels are elevated, his tube feeding may need to be altered to a lower level of carbohydrate to decrease CO_2 waste. It was stated that he seems to calm when being held and particularly enjoys being wrapped tightly. These techniques can particularly be used to avoid agitation, thus lower oxygen consumption. It will also be important to control his fever should he develop an infection since fever not only increases oxygen consumption but increases CO_2 levels.

B.   **As a newborn, you would be most concerned if TJ developed a respiratory rate of >_____ .**

C.   **Why is tachypnea a priority assessment in the very young? In addition to rate, what other nursing assessments are important in this age group?**

A rate of > 40. Tachypnea is often the first sign of respiratory distress in the very young and is associated with an increase in work of breathing. Other important assessments include: assessing for nasal flaring, intercostal and/or substernal retractions, rhythm, presence of adventitious breath sounds, respiratory effort, and arterial blood gases

C.   **The module lists criteria used in children to discriminate between two types of respiratory failure: Type I and Type II. Which does TJ have? Is it consistent with the probable diagnosis?**

He should have Type I, which is characteristic of atelectasis and pulmonary edema, with its primary problem of low PaO_2. We know that hypoxemia is a problem in TJ since he decompensates frequently and is requiring PEEP on the ventilator. He also fits the description of Type II because of an obstructive component to his disorder. This is characterized by his increased PCO_2 levels. TJ's situation demonstrates that classification systems, while useful as guides, may not adequately reflect reality in complex situations.

II.   PERFUSION

TJ's blood pressure is 82/58, his pulse is 168 and respirations are 64/minute. At 3 days post birth, his ductus arteriosus opened.

A.   **What is the clinical significance of his patent ductus arteriosus?**
The patent ductus arteriosus will increase his hypoxemia due to mixing of pulmonary and systemic blood. The degree of mixing will impact on the severity of hypoxemia. Clinically, he would show signs of hypoxemia (increased BP, P, R, decreased PaO_2 and decreased SaO_2..

B.   **Examine TJ's blood pressure and pulse and respirations. Interpret these values based on his age.**
P = 168. As a newborn, TJ/s pulse is within normal limits (120-180/minute). You would anticipate and increase in rate rather than an increase in contractility or change in preload and afterload in a newborn.
BP = 82/58. TJ's systolic BP is below the normal range for his age (neonate = SBP 85-100 with a DBP 51-65. His cardiomegaly may cause a decrease in cardiac output. Cardiac output is also decreased by positive pressure ventilation as well as positive end expiratory pressure (PEEP).
R = 64. TJ is experiencing tachypnea. Normally his rate should be below 40/minute. Tachypnea of > 60/minute is considered clinically significant respiratory distress. His rate may be partially due to compensatory mechanisms to increase his tissue oxygenation.

C.   **Is there evidence of decreased peripheral tissue perfusion?**
Other than TJ's intermittent cyanosis, there are no data given in the scenario to support this, though he is at risk for this problem. Students could be asked what type of assessments would they want to perform to assess this further.

III.   FLUIDS

A.   **The nurse is assessing for the signs of dehydration in TJ. What would be assessed in a neonate?**
Refer to Table 32-26, p. 591 - Clinical Assessment Data: Degrees of Dehydration

B.   **What kind of intravenous solution support would you anticipate to help maintain TJ's perfusion?**
If his BP continues to drop, his fluid administration might include normal saline or lactated Ringer's solution of 20 mL/kg. At approximately 2 Kg in weight, TJ would receive about 40 mL of IV fluid.

C.   **If TJ weighs approximately 2 Kg, his daily maintenance fluid needs would be _____mL.**

Using the calculation in Table 32-25, p. 590, his fluid needs would be 200 mL per 24 hours. This would be calculated as: 100 mL x 2 Kg = 200 mL/24 hours

D. **What interventions can the nurse take to reduce TJ's risk of infection?**

Refer to Table 32-33, p. 600. Preventive measures and early detection should be emphasized. Table 32-32, p. 600 lists a variety of assessments that are associated with immunocompetence problems in the young.

[If there is sufficient time, the teacher might want to explore the psychosocial aspects of this problem (i.e. the parent's fears, financial implications, etc.]

Case Study
The Case of Amanda
A Child with Multiple Problems

DIRECTIONS:

The Case of Amanda is an optional case study that provides multiple possible focuses both physiologic, ethical, and psychosocial. It is suggested that the teacher develop study questions based on desired emphasis.

****

Amanda is a 10 year old girl who was admitted on July 29th of this year. Her admission diagnosis was: Renal failure; Transplant.

Present Health Status

Amanda has experienced renal failure for eight years. She has been on CAPD (Continuous Ambulatory Peritoneal Dialysis) for three years. A cadaver transplant was unsuccessful last year. She is now being admitted for a second transplant attempt.

Personal/Social History

Amanda and a younger brother have lived in a foster home with several other children for three years. She continues to have infrequent contact with her biological parents. She ha a close relationship with her brother and has strong emotional ties with her biological parents. The plan is for permanent foster care, as adoptive placement of both children together is unlikely. Amanda attends a multiply handicapped class. She is considered trainably mentally handicapped and functions at K to 1 grade level. School attendance has been variable due to many health problems. Her low energy level also interferes with her performance. Amanda is fearful of the transplant, particularly in relation to pain and rejection. Amanda receives no income, relying only on health insurance via Medicaid.

PAST HEALTH HISTORY

Amanda was born with a mylomeningocele at the T-11 level. It was repaired at four days without complications. She had a V-P shunt placed at two weeks. To date, she has had thirteen surgeries (six in the past two years) and multiple hospitalizations for orthopedic bracing, shunt infections and revisions (she currently has a V-A shunt), UTI's, tinchoff placement, and difficulties with peritoneal dialysis, including repeated peritonitis. Most recent hospitalization was 4 months ago to remove a necrotic donor kidney. She is being followed by the outpatient clinics for the following problems:

Renal failure, herpes (opthamologic, opportunistic infection from immunosuppressant therapy), hypo-thyroidism, V-A shunt, leg bracing, psychiatry for separation from family and catastrophic illness, and general care through pediatrics.

Present Medications Taken at Home

Rocaltrol	0.25 mg every day
$FeSO_4$	300 mg BID
Nephrocaps	1 every day
Alucap	2 every day
Synthroid	75 mcg/day
Viroptic	1 gtt every 2 hours
Macrodantin	50 mg TID

PRN Medications: Atenolol for diastolic BP of > 100 mmHg
Kaexolate for K+ > 6

Family History

Maternal: Drug abuse

Paternal: Drug abuse
Siblings: two live with parents -- both are low functioning. Two had myelomingocele and died.
Another brother has myelomingocele and is living in foster home.
Parents are first cousins and low functioning.

INITIAL NURSING ASSESSMENT

VS: BP = 98/64, P = 100/minute, R = 16, T = 98.2 (O)
Weight = 70 pounds, Height = 49.5 inches

Neurologic: Responsive but lethargic. Verbalizes without difficulty but tends not to voice complaints. V-A shunt palpable. No evidence of increased intracranial pressure. Gets headache and is more lethargic when ICP increases. Has decreased sensation to mid-thigh and no sensation below that point.

Respiratory: Breath sounds are equal and clear and unlabored.

Cardiovascular: Feet are slightly cool, edematous and cyanotic. Pedal pulses are thready but equal bilaterally. slow capillary refill in feet but <2 seconds in hands. Pulse is strong and regular.

Gastrointestinal: Amanda is anorexic. She has been on Travesorb Renal NG feedings at night since last fall (480 mL at night per pump). She is on a moderate sodium restricted diet. All teeth are present and in good condition. Her abdomen is round and soft with multiple scars. She has a tinchoff catheter in place with no drainage or skin breakdown around the site. Bowel sounds are normoactive in all four quadrants.

Musculoskeletal: Amanda can move her arms equally and without difficulty. She moves her hips well. There is little movement below her hips. She is able to ambulate short distances with crutches and braces. She is able to put her braces on herself. She does little physical activity due to fatigue.

Genitourinary: Amanda is in Stage 3 of sexual maturation. Her menses have not yet begun. She has received instruction regarding it at home.

Psychosocial: Amanda's foster mother is an RN. Amanda is kept neatly groomed and is dressed appropriate for age. She is independent with minimal assistance for her ADLs. She has visions about imminent death and voices a sense of peace about this. She has had counseling with her minister and Psychiatry. She relies on her foster mother for daily support.

MEDICAL TEAM FINDINGS AND PROGRESS NOTES

Admitted for renal transplant. Her condition is stable on peritoneal dialysis.

CURRENT ABNORMAL LABS REPORTS
pH	7.31
Hct	22
BUN	100
K+	5.5

CURRENT MEDICAL ORDERS
1. D_5W at keep vein open rate
2. Pre-Op scrub
3. NPO
4. CBC with diff, Astra-9, Hitachi
5. [No medication orders at this time due to impending surgery]

OVERHEAD TRANSPARENCY MASTERS

Overhead Transparency Masters

Figure   5 - 1   Components of ventilation.

Figure   5 - 8   Comparison of ventilatory modes.

Figure   7 - 1   Three components of oxygenation.

Figure   9 - 4   Mechanism of MODS.

Figure 12 - 12   Ventricular function curve.

Figure 13 - 1   Membrane permeability changes in nonpacemaker myocardial cells.

Figure 13 - 30   A pacemaker in DDD mode is capable of exhibiting any of four pacing patterns, all within a brief period of time.

Figure 15 - 4   Location of intracranial pressure monitors.

Figure 16 - 3   Cerebral blood flow thresholds in focal ischemia.

Figure 16 - 5   The ischemic cascade.

Figure 18 - 3   Schematic representation of the physical effects of spinal cord injury. (*From Somers, M.F. [1992]. Spinal cord injury: Functional rehabilitation. Norwalk, CT: Appleton & Lange.*)

Figure 24 - 1   Consequences of insulin deficit.

Figure 26 - 4   Nephron transport. (*From Ulrich, B.T. [1989]. Nephrology nursing: Concepts and strategies, p. 15. Norwalk, CT: Appleton & Lange.*)

Figure 26 - 5   The renin–angiotensin system. (*From Ulrich, B.T. [1989]. Nephrology nursing: Concepts and strategies, p. 22. Norwalk, CT: Appleton & Lange.*)

Figure 26 - 6   Three types of venous access. (*From Ahrens, T., and Prentice, D. [1993]. Critical care certification preparation and review, 3rd ed. Norwalk, CT: Appleton & Lange.*)

Figure 29 - 3   Changes in capillary permeability determine extravascular fluid levels.

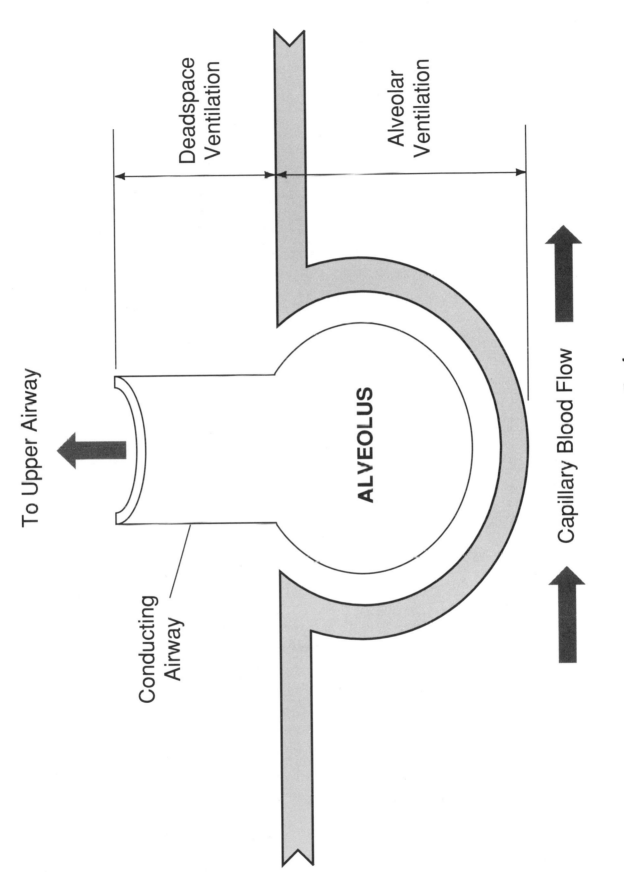

Figure 5 - 1

From: Kidd & Wagner: *High Acuity Nursing,* **2nd e**

© 1997 by Appleton & Lange

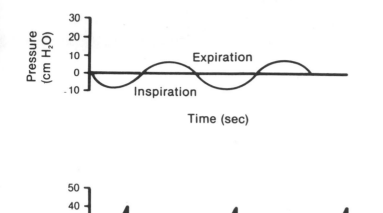

Spontaneous Breathing

Patient has full work of breathing: determining rate, V_T, and rhythm.

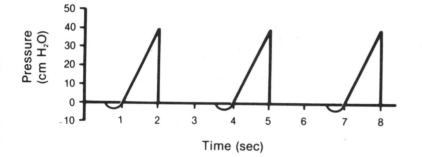

Controlled Ventilation

Patient has no work breathing: ventilator will rhythmically deliver V_T at preset rate.

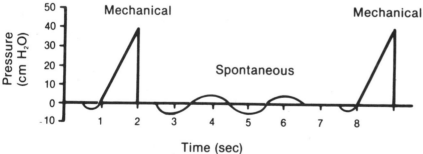

Assist-Control

Patient has minimal work of breathing during initial expansion of chest, then ventilator will deliver preset V_T.

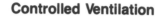

Intermittent Mandatory Ventilation (IMV)

Patient has a variable work of breathing: the mandatory ventilated breaths occur at a preset rate and V_T, but the patient may take spontaneous breaths between the machine-delivered breaths.

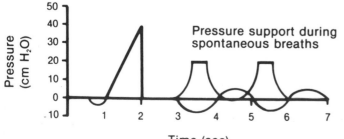

IMV with Pressure Support (12 cm H_2O)

Patient has low-to-moderate work of breathing: the spontaneous breaths are supported with a preset pressure assistance.

Figure 5-8

From: Kidd & Wagner: *High Acuity Nursing*, 2nd ed.

© 1997 by Appleton & Lange

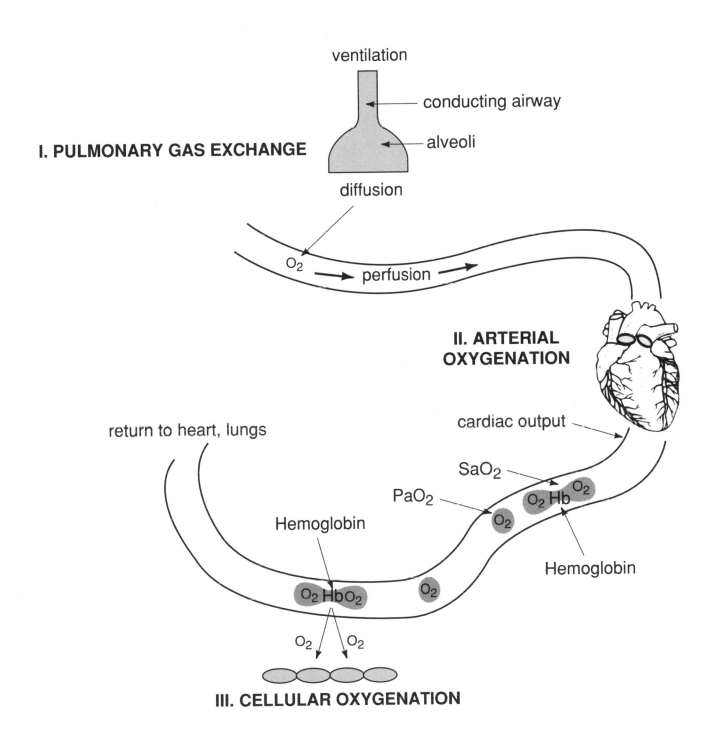

Figure 7 - 1

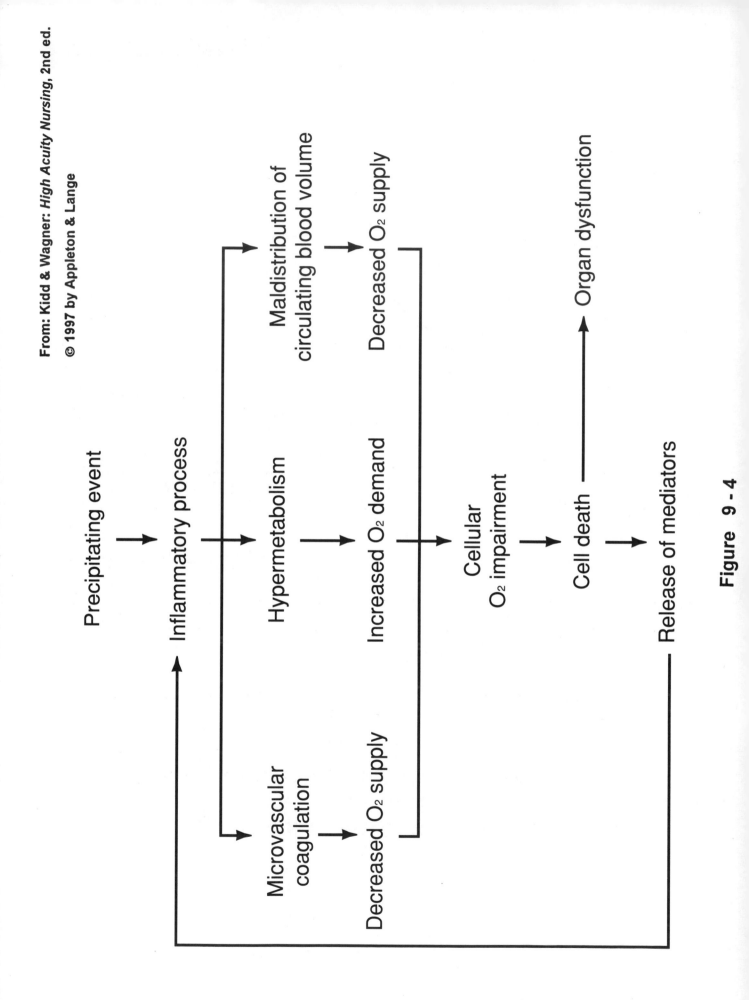

Figure 9 - 4

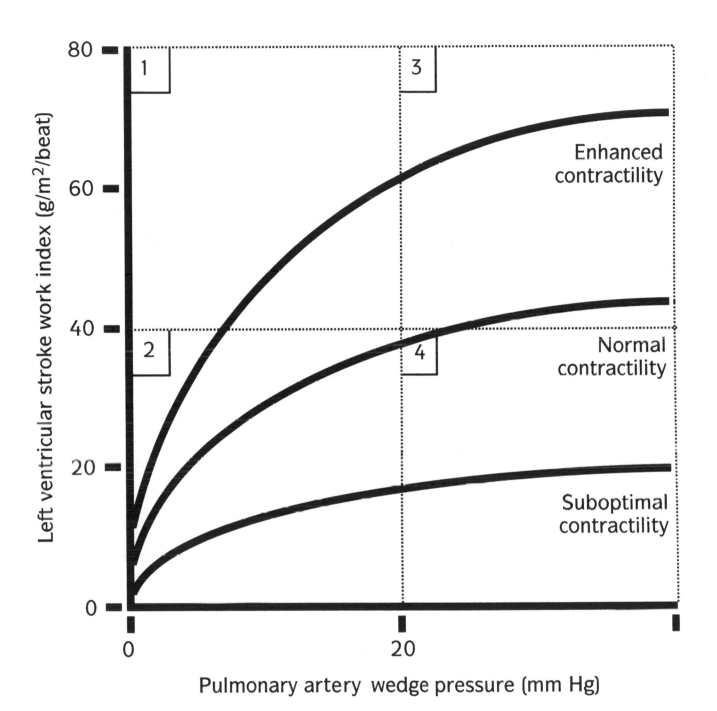

Quadrant 1: Optimal function; Quadrant 2: Hypovolemia;
Quadrant 3: Hypervolemia; Quadrant 4: Cardiac failure

Figure 12 - 12

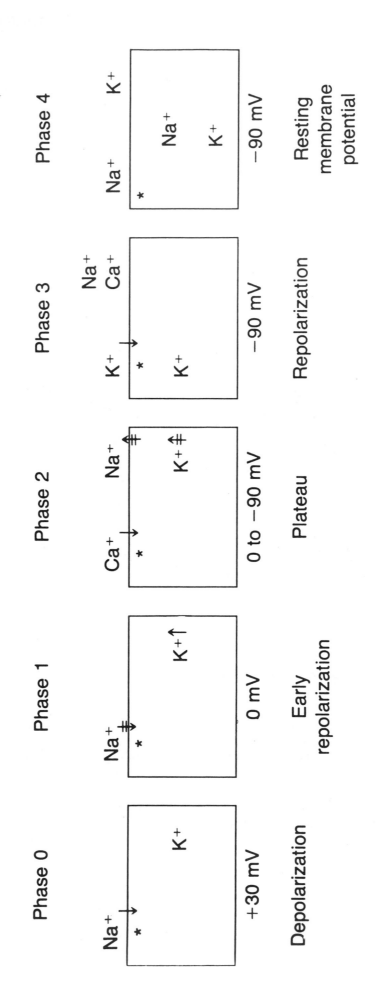

Figure 13 - 1

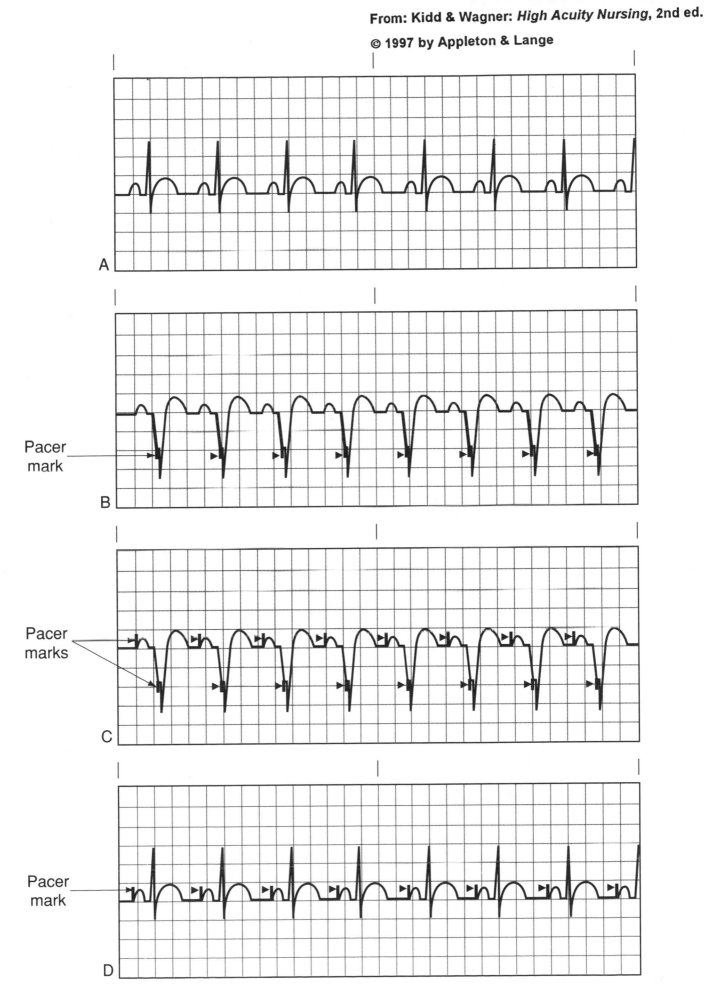

A

Pacer
mark

B

Pacer
marks

C

Pacer
mark

D

Figure 13 - 30

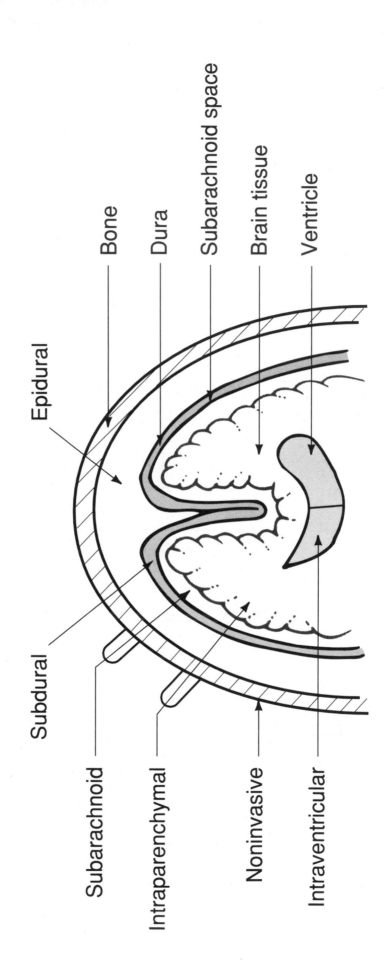

Epidural

Bone

Dura

Subarachnoid space

Brain tissue

Ventricle

Subdural

Subarachnoid

Intraparenchymal

Noninvasive

Intraventricular

Figure 15 - 4

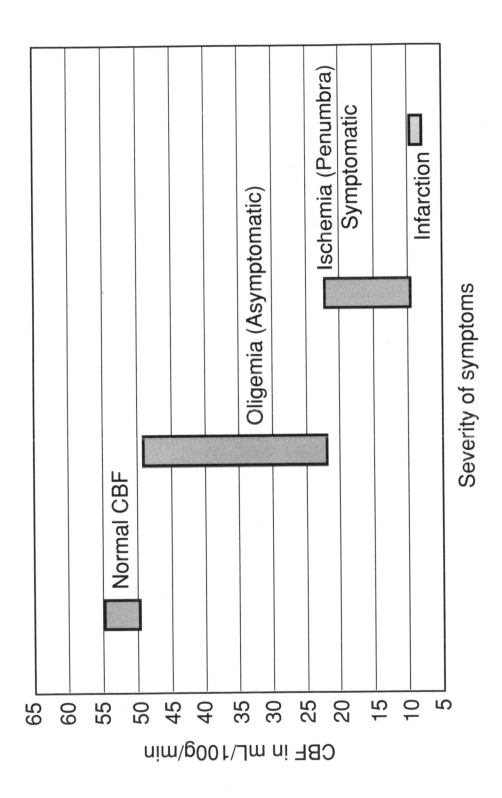

Figure 16 - 3

A. Pump failure, leading to anerobic metabolism, leading to cellular acidosis

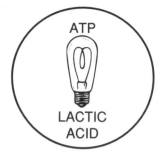

B. Ionic imbalances: cellular edema.

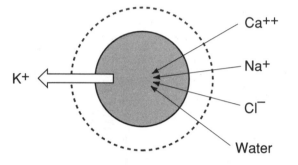

C. Intracellular accumulation of calcium and glutamate's role.

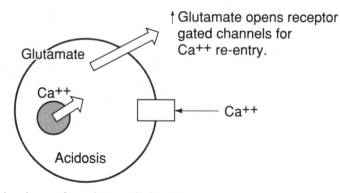

Ca++ release from intracellular stores
Glutamate release Cerebral blood flow
<20 mL/100 g • min

D. Cellular degradation.

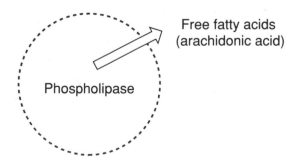

Phospholipases activated by excess Ca++,
promote breakdown of cellular membrane,
degrading cellular DNA and its proteins

Figure 16 - 5

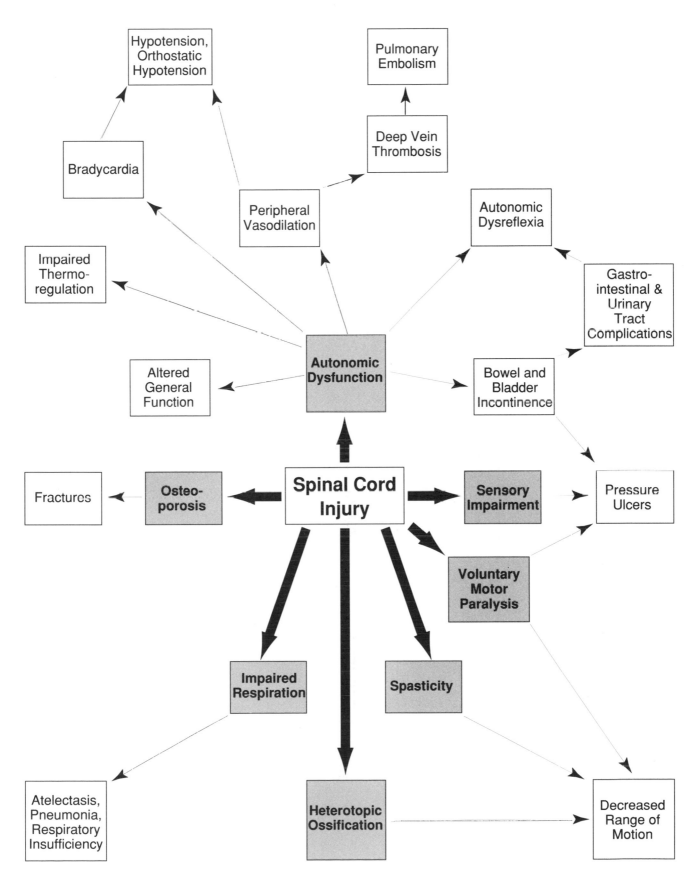

Figure 18 - 3

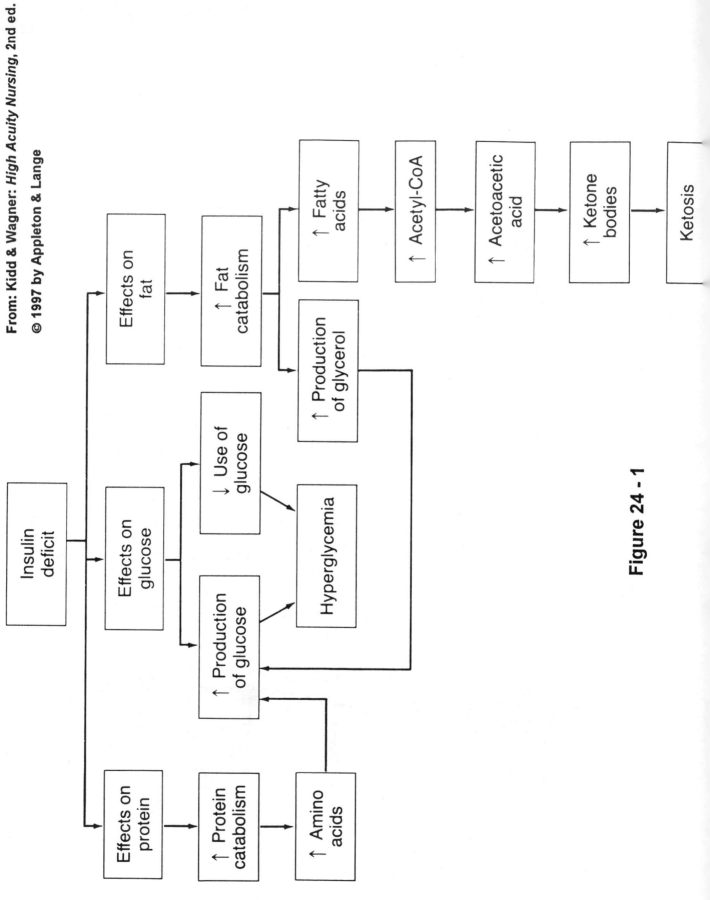

Figure 24 - 1

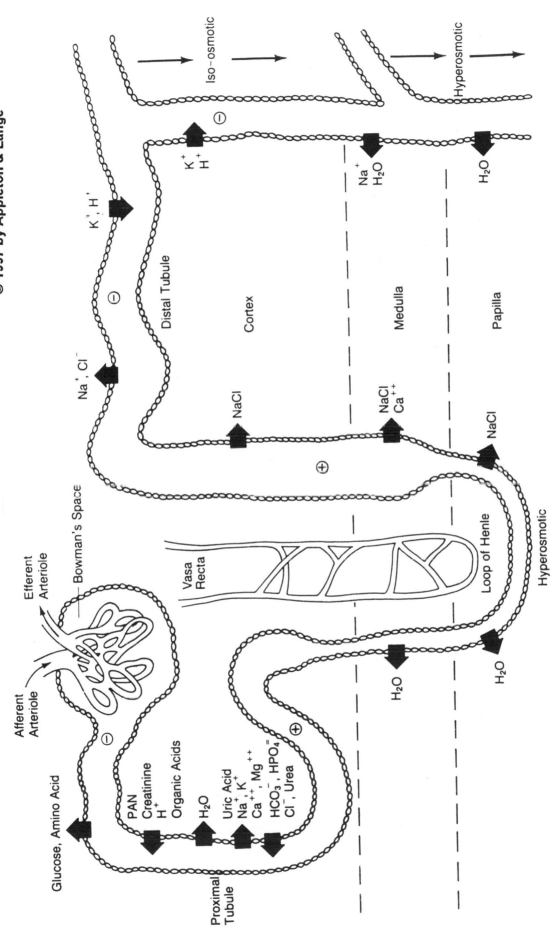
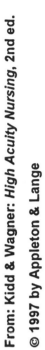

Figure 26 - 4

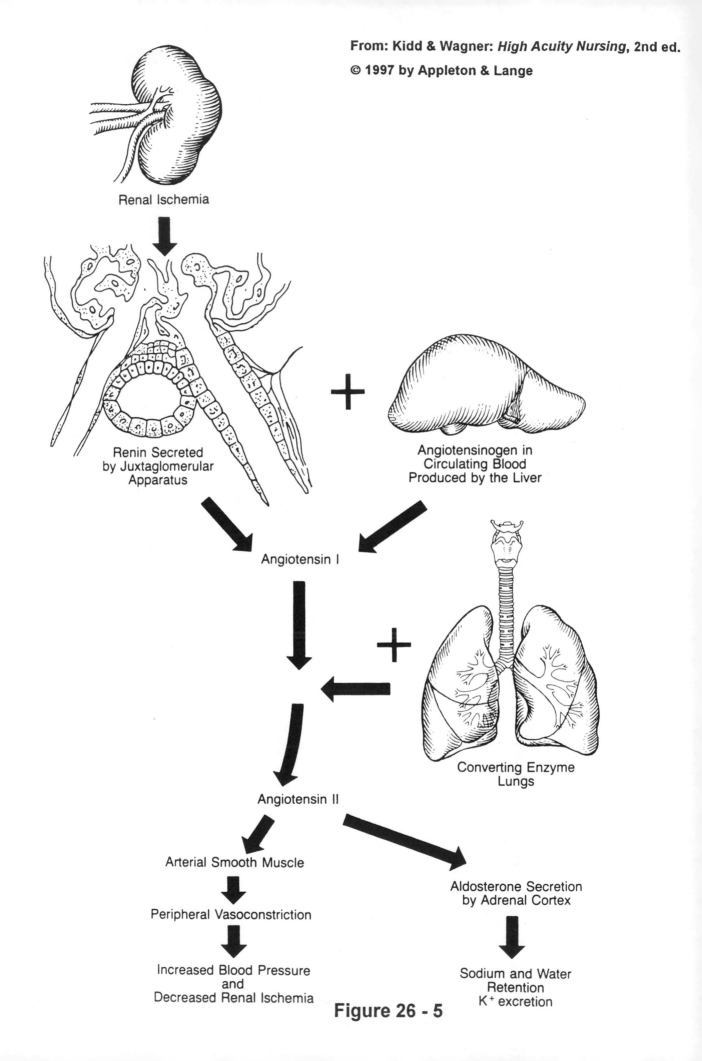

Renal Ischemia

Renin Secreted
by Juxtaglomerular
Apparatus

+

Angiotensinogen in
Circulating Blood
Produced by the Liver

Angiotensin I

+

Converting Enzyme
Lungs

Angiotensin II

Arterial Smooth Muscle

Peripheral Vasoconstriction

Increased Blood Pressure
and
Decreased Renal Ischemia

Aldosterone Secretion
by Adrenal Cortex

Sodium and Water
Retention
K^+ excretion

Figure 26 - 5

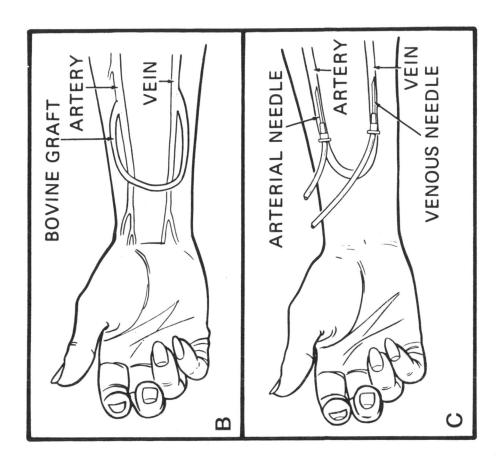

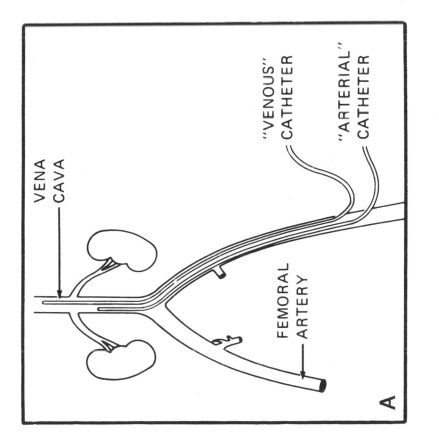

Figure 26 - 6

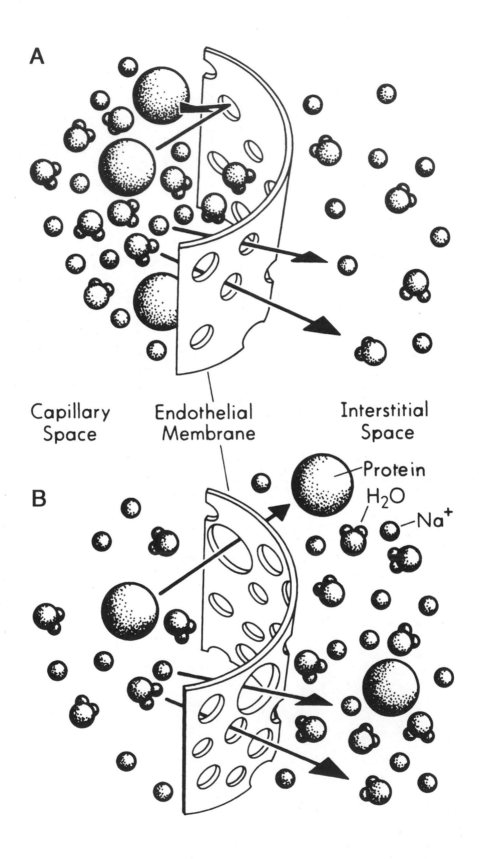

Figure 29 - 3